The Unwelcome Companion

Rick Fowler's book is a moving description of what it feels like to have TS and associated disorders...entertaining, informative, and well written.

Tourette Gazette, Washington DC, Maryland, and Virginia Winter 1996

It should be a helpful book for patients and their families to read. As far as I know it is the first of its kind. Nicely written, very clear.

Ruth Dowling Bruun, MD.

Clinical Associate Professor of Psychiatry at Cornell University Medical School, co-author of *A Mind of Its Own, Tourette Syndrome: A Story and A Guide*

Readers are provided with a compelling narrative of the symptoms, sensations, and what it is like to cope with TS on an everyday basis...Well researched.

Tourette Syndrome Association, Inc. National Newsletter

A good read! Surely expands understanding of TS.

Tourette Syndrome Association of Pennsylvania

In general, books about medical or psychological topics prove extremely boring and tedious to the non-professional reader. Not so with The Unwelcome Companion...easy to read and absorbing...the perfect measure of medical information (in understandable laymen's terms) and personal experience...

The Times-Georgian

The Unwelcome Companion
An Insider's View of Tourette Syndrome
Revised Edition

Rick Fowler

Silver Run Publications, Inc.
Cashiers, NC
1996

The Unwelcome Companion
An Insider's View of Tourette Syndrome
Revised Edition

published by
Silver Run Publications, Inc.
P.O. Box 55
Cashiers, NC 28717 USA

Copyright 1995–original edition
© 1996–revised edition
by Rick Fowler

ISBN # 0-9646376-9-3
Library of Congress Catalog Card Number
96-68438

Edited by
Johnny Reynolds and Jennifer E. McKee
Cover art by Vanessa Weaver

printed in the United States of America

Acknowledgements

I could not have written this book without the help of numerous individuals. I greatly appreciate their assistance, guidance, and patience.

For medical advice, either personal or technical, I thank Lee Stringfellow, M.D. and staff, M.L. Johnson, M.D., Dr. Cindy Darden, Dr. Manfred Mueller, homeopathic physician, Joseph White, M.D., David M. Wheeler, M.D., Neal Priest, M.D., and Dr. Pat Priest. I would also like to thank Mark Zachary, family pharmacist, for proofing and comments in chapter eight.

Special thanks to Sue Levy of the Tourette Syndrome Association, Inc. for her valuable guidance, and to Dr. Ruth Dowling Bruun, M.D. for her wonderful advice and support. To Hope Press and David E. Comings, M.D., thank-you for the use of the excerpt from *Don't Think About Monkeys*, which appears in chapter five. Thanks to Cynthia Weaver and the Pilot Club of Athens, GA.

Thanks to the following people for editing, suggestions, and proofreading: Suzanne Edwards, Anita Blaschak, Clint and Joanne Edwards, Jill Leite, Paula Gordon, and especially my editors, Jennifer McKee and Johnny Reynolds. Thanks to Norbert Miller and Vanessa Weaver for artistic guidance.

On a more personal note, I would like to express my gratitude to my family for their endless support over the years, and to Anita Blaschak and Debbie Norton for suggesting that I undertake this endeavor. I would also like to express my appreciation to Lyndon McKee, who lent enormous editorial support and encouragement throughout the course of this project. To Sharon Johnson: Thanks for your wisdom, and for shining the light of hope to guide me.

Very special thanks and all my love to Sherry Joyce Johnson for being there, putting up with me, sticking by me during my periods of frustration, and loving me unconditionally. Without your editorial assistance and emotional support, I could not have finished this book.

DISCLAIMER

This book is designed to provide information with regard to the subject matter covered. It is written with the understanding that the publisher and author are not engaged in rendering medical, psychological, legal, or other professional services to the reader. If medical, legal, or other assistance is required, the services of a competent professional in the appropriate field should be sought.

Although the author is not a physician, all medical, pharmacological, and psychiatric information contained within the text has been thoroughly checked for accuracy by medical professionals. However, there may be mistakes, both typographical and in content. Therefore this text should be used as a general guide, and not as the ultimate source of information concerning Tourette syndrome or any other medical disorder. Furthermore, this book contains information only up to the date of publication.

Personal information about the author, where included, is for educational purposes only. The author makes no claim that such experiences are universal. Therefore, he is neither discouraging nor recommending any treatment, medication, or therapy discussed in this book.

Neither the author nor the publisher shall have or accept any liability or responsibility to any person or entity with respect to loss or damage or any other problem caused, or alleged to be caused, directly or indirectly by the information contained in this book.

Contents

When I breathe, it breathes. When I speak, it speaks. When I try to sleep, it won't let me. Whatever I attempt to do, it's there...waiting to spoil the moment. To a doctor, it's a disorder, a medical oddity. To an onlooker, it's a spectacle—perhaps humorous, perhaps grotesque. To me, it's a monster, a demon, a hellish beast who has no right to exist in my world or anyone else's—it's my unwelcome companion.

A percentage of the profits from the sale of this book will be donated to The Tourette Syndrome Association, Inc.

The Unwelcome Companion

An Insider's View of Tourette Syndrome

Introduction

It was two o'clock on a Saturday morning. I looked out from the stage and saw the reflection of dim exit lights across a scuffed floor. The club's employees were beginning to clean tables, and the last of the crowd was finally milling out the door. I was both tired and elated, for tonight's set had been a long, but good one. There had been a sizable crowd and the band had played well, inspired by an enthusiastic audience.

As I put away my guitar and prepared to leave the stage, our vocalist walked up laughing. The club owner had just told her that he enjoyed the music, but was concerned about the guitar player's "obvious" drug problem. She giggled, "This guy thinks that you're some kind of addict in need of a fix. He claims he knows a doper when he sees one, and the way you jerk around is a sure sign." She rolled her eyes. "I tried to explain, but he wouldn't listen. He kept saying that your drug problem would do nothing but drag our band down."

My elation instantly evaporated. The band members may find these misunderstandings amusing, but tonight's incident really bothered me. After years of dealing with similar negative reactions to my twitches and unusual movements, I was beginning to wear thin.

The club owner was right about one thing—I do have a problem. But my odd behavior is not caused by illegal drug use. It results from a neurological disorder called Tourette syndrome (TS).

Though originally identified in the 1800's, this mysterious illness somehow slipped through the pages of medical journals until the late 1960's. Physicians and psychologists knew virtually nothing about TS, which was considered to be an extreme oddity.

Until recently most people who had the disorder, characterized by involuntary movements and vocal outbursts, were thought to be insane. They were typically locked away in mental hospitals, given heavy doses of tranquilizing drugs, subjected to electroshock therapy, or in rare instances, given lobotomies.

Others, whose families came from superstitious backgrounds, were thought to be possessed by demons, and subjected to ritualistic exorcisms. At one point, this was such a common occurrence that Tourette syndrome eventually came to be described by psychiatrists as "the medical cause of possession."[1]

Throughout history, TS has been distorted by myth, and inadequately defined in medical literature. It continues to be misunderstood today. Children with the disorder are sometimes punished for their bizarre actions, and are perceived to be either mischievous or mentally disturbed. Adults are ostracized for their inappropriate behaviors, and may experience difficulty holding jobs or developing successful social relationships.

Fortunately, there has been increased discussion of TS in recent years, and several excellent publications on the topic are now available. Most are written by physicians and researchers who have either treated or conducted studies of Tourette patients.

In spite of this wealth of information, many people, including some medical professionals, still have an inaccurate view of the internal mental processes which induce the behaviors associated with TS. Such ambiguous perceptions can make it difficult for doctors to relate to and treat patients with this syndrome.

For this reason, I feel that it is important to present a view from within the patient's mind—a view which provides the reader with a first hand account of the nature and intensity of the battle which rages inside the Tourettic brain.

When I first decided to write this book, my biggest fear was that readers would think I was complaining or seeking sympathy. This is not the purpose of *The Unwelcome Companion.* I grew up with a wonderful family and many caring friends. I have only a moderate case of TS, which allows me to function reasonably well, and I have little to complain about.

There are those who are not so lucky. Some are totally debilitated by Tourette syndrome. Others have no love and support from the people around them. They must face both the torturous symptoms of their illness and the damaging curse of being rejected by those nearest to them. Still others live in communities where the doctors remain unfamiliar with TS. These patients may never discover the origin of their devastating symptoms.

In my travels, I have happened upon a few such unfortunate souls, and have heard their stories. Some have been disowned by family members, fired from jobs, or expelled from schools. Many vaguely recall lost childhoods, their memories and dreams destroyed by the long-term use of inappropriately prescribed medications.

Perhaps such injustices would not occur if there were a broader understanding of Tourette syndrome. Although there is no known cure for the disorder, in many cases proper medical care can calm the symptoms. Understanding can accomplish even more, by preventing much of the humiliation, rejection, and resulting emotional damage associated with Tourette syndrome—damage which can cause a person to become withdrawn, depressed, and unable to function in society.

The emotional and physical trauma of Tourette syndrome makes it one of the most disruptive disorders in existence. It upsets every aspect of a person's life, public and private, as well as the lives of peers, relatives, teachers, employers, and co-workers. They too must face the awkward task of dealing with the constant distraction, interruption, and embarrassment caused by tics.

People who have Tourette syndrome not only reveal their disorder, they unwillingly broadcast it. Onlookers watch helplessly as this curse twists and jerks its hostage into a contorted spectacle. The affliction makes its presence known almost as if it is proud, boastful of a nature which defies every civilized behavior known to humankind. It tries to consume the sufferer, exposing not the grace of the individual, but the impediment of disease.

Chapter one
It Was Not Insanity!

Hospital waiting rooms sometimes seem brilliantly designed to intimidate visitors. The smell of antiseptic potions, the sound of muffled voices discussing life and death problems, and the fear of nearby airborne viruses can be extremely upsetting.

As patients tentatively look around the room, they share similar thoughts. In addition to worrying about their own problems, they are curious about each other's diseases, and the possibility of contracting them. A general uneasiness hangs in the air.

It was in such a place that I found myself, waiting uncomfortably with dozens of other patients, one summer afternoon in 1974. One by one, we were called in to the examining rooms to be prodded, tested, and tortured.

Some of us had already been through the probing and were anxiously awaiting the results of our examinations. At this point, I had been in the hospital building for at least seven hours; I was ready to go home.

Although my tests were not particularly painful, the wait was excruciating. It was not possible for me to sit quietly and patiently. I was constantly moving my hands and feet, clearing my throat, and shifting around in my seat in a futile attempt to get comfortable. However, my discomfort went far beyond the hardness of a waiting room chair.

I was never able to sit still, even in the best of chairs. I could not rest in any position without having to endure the constant involuntary movements of my arms, legs, and facial muscles. I had difficulty speaking without repeatedly clearing my throat or grunting. True relaxation was something so remote that I had no recollection of how it could possibly feel. This "nervous problem" was the reason I was here—and at this point, it was coming on full-throttle.

I was acutely aware of the stares of others as I fought the uncontrollable jerks of my neck and arms. The more I fought them, the more persistent and urgent they became. I felt like a freak on display.

As I continued my struggle against these contortions, I began to recall the years of endless battle with this condition. By now, I had seen at least a dozen doctors, and had been tested and treated unsuccessfully for any number of diseases. My parents had reached their wit's end. This time, I was having a complete physical examination at a hospital with impeccable credentials.

I had actually looked forward to this day, excited by the possibility of finally learning the nature of my problem. Maybe it could be treated. Maybe I could stop taking one ineffective prescription drug after another. I was tired of the side effects of these drugs and the withdrawal symptoms which resulted from switching medications every few months. Although I was barely in my twenties, I had already taken more prescription drugs than anyone I had ever known—more than many people consume in a lifetime.

It was a relief when at long last my name was called, and I went in to see the team of doctors who had completed my extensive physical examination. I would finally know what was causing these strange symptoms.

There were five or six doctors and a couple of other medical professionals in the consultation room. They all seemed to look at me as if I had wasted their time.

"Son, we've checked everything we can think of,"

the chief doctor said. "There's nothing that we can find physically wrong with you. You just need to calm down."

In disbelief, I asked, "What causes me to jerk around? Why does my arm flip up? Why am I always blinking my eyes? Isn't there some reason for this?"

The doctor replied, "There is no physical cause; maybe you're just nervous. You should consider talking to a counselor. The problem is in your head, nothing more."

This verdict was crushing. I had truly hoped for some kind of answer this time. Was I really crazy? I did not think so, yet the tests had shown no physical reason for my behavior. I began to get angry with the doctors for failing, frustrated with myself for not being able to control my behavior, and ashamed of being so messed up in the head.

For the next several years, I continued to search for another explanation. I felt that I was reasonably well-adjusted, had a clear understanding of reality, and was able to think in a rational manner, even during my so-called "fits." In my opinion, that ruled out the possibility that the symptoms resulted from a severe psychological disturbance.

During my search, various doctors tried to figure out what was causing me to jerk around so strangely.

No one could find a clue. I became increasingly depressed with every stranger's stare, every curious person's comment, and every doctor's failed diagnosis.

Finally, one day, a friend mentioned a magazine article he had read about a disorder of the central nervous system called *Tourette syndrome.* He felt that the symptoms described in this article fit my condition. I had never heard of such an illness, especially not one which causes people to shout profanity. Nevertheless, the motor symptoms he described sounded remarkably familiar, and I felt that it was worth checking into.

I made yet another appointment and discussed the possibility with my family doctor, a dedicated, compassionate physician who seemed frustrated that, over the years, he had been unable to diagnose my condition. Like most family practitioners at the time, he knew nothing about Tourette syndrome, so he referred me to a neurologist.

The neurologist immediately confirmed my suspicions. He went on to explain that TS is a neurological disorder in which the patient exhibits uncontrollable movements of various muscle groups, and utters sounds or vocal outbursts. Its severity may range from mere aggravation to complete debilitation. In approximately one-fourth of cases, the symptoms include the unintentional shouting of offensive or obscene statements.

Other signs of the disorder include the repeating of others' words or actions, and obsessive-compulsive rituals (such as repeatedly touching people or objects, or checking things over and over). Short attention span and hyperactivity are also common among the vast array of symptoms, as are learning disabilities, inappropriate or self-destructive behaviors, and depression.[2]

At first, I was shocked to learn that other people also had this disorder. I had always thought that I was the only person in the world who was fighting this battle. That doctors have actually treated thousands of patients with similar symptoms seemed unbelievable to me. What a relief it was to learn that I was not alone, that this strange disorder had a name, and that it was not *insanity!*

Chapter two
A Misunderstood Disorder

The first documented evidence of Tourette syndrome appeared in medical literature in 1825, although at the time, the disease did not have a name. The patient in question was the Marquise de Dampierre, a French noblewoman. Her symptoms included most of the abnormal behaviors now associated with this disorder. She would violently move and jerk parts of her body, repeat statements or sounds made by others in an echoing fashion, and blurt out offensive and often profane phrases. In spite of her grotesque behavior, this woman was otherwise considered to be intelligent and sane.

Years later, a French neurologist, Georges Gilles de la Tourette, became fascinated by a disorder in which those afflicted exhibited uncontrollable "tics." In 1885, he studied and described to the medical community

16

nine cases of this strange set of symptoms, or "syndrome." The doctor personally examined six of the patients, including the Marquise de Dampierre, who was by this time an elderly woman.

In each case, symptoms included *motor tics* (involuntary gestures and movements of the extremities, torso, and facial muscles) and *vocal tics,* such as grunting sounds, barks, yelps, and the occasional shouting of profanity. Many of the patients were troubled with obsessive thoughts and compulsive behavior patterns. Some would repeatedly perform grooming tasks, while others touched objects over and over. In spite of these odd behaviors, all patients seemed mentally sound.

As a result of Dr. Gilles de la Tourette's studies, the disorder became known as *Gilles de la Tourette syndrome,* or the shorter version, *Tourette syndrome.* It is also referred to as *Tourette's disorder, Tourette's syndrome,* or simply *TS.*

Misunderstanding has plagued Tourette syndrome sufferers since long before the disorder had a name. In the past, people who made strange noises or bizarre gestures were usually thought to be either mentally unstable, completely insane, or possessed by demons. Although demonic possession seems an outlandish diagnosis today, how else could an eighteenth-century physician or clergyman have explained reprehensible remarks and gestures from otherwise sane people? These inappropriate, uncontrollable actions surely must have been the work of the devil.

It is now known that Tourette syndrome is a neurological disorder, not a mental illness or a manifestation of demonic possession. The condition is inherited, and is caused by neurochemical malfunction, not deep-rooted psychological problems or spiritual takeover.

Nevertheless, well-meaning but misinformed psychologists continue to erroneously assume that symptoms result from a patient's hidden hatred for a parent, suppressed memories of abuse, a desperate need for attention, or some other environmental stressor. Failed attempts at psychotherapy frequently cause feelings of confusion, guilt, and frustration, yet repeatedly prove to be of little or no value in curing tics. [3]

In many cases, a child with Tourette syndrome will start to show the first symptoms during a stressful period. This connection between stressful events and the onset of tics may cause others to mistake the symptoms for a reaction to a tense situation. The circumstances may differ, but the scenario frequently involves a series of erroneous conclusions.

For instance, a child enters a new school. Shortly thereafter, he begins to blink his eyes rapidly and utter grunting sounds. These actions are initially viewed as attention-grabbing devices. As the disorder takes its course, the symptoms worsen. The child, teased by other children, and tormented by the internal tension of TS, begins to develop aggressive tendencies and difficulty getting along with classmates. He is soon branded as a problem child. His parents take him to a counselor, who assumes that his behavior is nothing more than a psychological reaction to the stress of the new school.

The child is, in fact, beginning to show signs of an inevitable biological disorder which has nothing to do with the new school. Any stressful circumstance could have lowered the child's defenses, triggering an on-slaught of his first symptoms of Tourette syndrome.

Unfortunately, similar situations often result in persecution of Tourettic children, not only by their peers, but by parents and teachers as well. Due to widespread ignorance, people with tics frequently become outcasts or subjects of ridicule. Their bizarre gestures and sounds are thought to be intentional, and are interpreted as deliberate acts of misbehavior. Under these circumstances, not only does the disorder go untreated, but it is compounded by feelings of guilt and low self-esteem.

Understanding on the part of parents, teachers, and physicians is an essential element in the management of TS. Only in recent years has the information to foster such understanding become available.

Medical reports published as late as 1982 declared that Tourette syndrome was "an extremely rare affliction." This is no longer considered to be true. Today, doctors estimate that as many as one in one hundred males, and one in three hundred females has TS—approximately two million people in the United States alone. As more doctors are learning to recognize and diagnose TS, these estimates will likely increase. Available statistics also fail to reflect the vast number of individuals with mild symptoms who never seek medical attention, and consequently remain undiagnosed.

One can only imagine the horror people with odd tics must have endured in days past. Untold numbers of fully cognizant, lucid people were locked away in asylums, subjected to barbaric rituals, or executed, their lives destroyed by nothing more than a disruptive and misunderstood neurological disorder.

Chapter three
Diagnosis of Tourette Syndrome

Gilles de la Tourette syndrome is unique among movement disorders. Although other neurological disorders, including *myoclonus, Huntington's disease, Sydenham's chorea,* and *Parkinson's disease,* may cause abnormal motor activity, the loss of coordination, jerks, or tremors associated with them bear little resemblance to the stereotyped tics of TS. Stereotyped movements are gestures which are repeated identically, as opposed to random twitches or tremors. This repetition is primarily what sets tic disorders apart.⁴

It is estimated that over one-fourth of all children may experience minor tics before adolescence, such as excessive eye blinking or repeated facial grimacing. Common childhood tics may vary in location and severity, and may last for years before disappearing.

Because they are not permanent, they are referred to as *Transient Tic Disorders.*

Another fairly common childhood condition is *Chronic Tic Disorder.* A chronic tic remains relatively unchanged throughout its duration, although it may also last for years.

When more than one tic occurs, the condition is called *Multiple Tic Disorder.* If several tics are present and remain constant in location and nature, *Chronic Multiple Tic Disorder* is indicated.

Some researchers feel that childhood tic disorders may be related to Tourette syndrome. Others feel that they are actually mild forms of the syndrome. Unfortunately, there is no easy way to distinguish the appearance of a child's temporary tic disorder from the onset of TS. Tics commonly begin to appear in children at around age seven, although they can show up as early as age three. If Tourette syndrome is indicated it usually becomes evident before age fifteen. If both motor and vocal tics occur before age twenty-one and persist for more than one year, a diagnosis of Tourette syndrome is likely.[5]

Related Disorders

Tourette syndrome is a complex disorder that can

mimic other disturbances, sometimes making accurate diagnosis difficult. It often includes an array of independent disorders, each of which can be disruptive or totally destructive to a person's well-being. It is not unusual for a doctor seeing a TS patient for the first time to notice only the associated disorder, failing to recognize Tourette syndrome as the root of the problem. These related disorders do not necessarily involve tics:

Hyperactivity literally means "over-activity," and is characterized by unusually high energy levels and excessive movement. A hyperactive child cannot sit still, is usually running or climbing, may have difficulty falling asleep, and is frequently a restless sleeper. Some of these symptoms may persist into adulthood.

Attention deficit disorder is a condition in which patients experience difficulty paying attention, are easily distracted, and frequently suffer severe learning problems. Impatience, excessive talking, inability to listen, and constant shifting from one activity to another are common in ADD.

Although most commonly seen in children, adults also suffer from hyperactivity, ADD, or both. *Attention deficit hyperactivity disorder* is a combination of the two. People with ADHD are usually fidgety and restless. They seem constantly on the go, frantic, and scattered. Quiet relaxation is generally impossible for these individuals; they must be moving about or talking constantly. ADHD sufferers are usually impulsive, irritable, and easily frustrated.

Varying degrees of ADHD are present in well over half of all TS patients, but most children who suffer from ADHD do not develop Tourette syndrome. It is difficult for a physician to predict TS in hyperactive children, as restlessness and other symptoms may be present for up to three years before any tics appear.

Obsessive-compulsive disorder is another condition which has been closely linked to TS. It can be debilitating, and like ADHD, can occur either independently or in conjunction with Tourette syndrome.

Obsessions are intrusive thoughts which constantly interrupt normal thinking patterns. These thoughts are sometimes unpleasant or morbid in nature, or may simply consist of a nonsensical phrase or mathematical process which plagues the mind. Obsessive-compulsive individuals are sometimes driven by extreme perfectionism, and constantly seek symmetry and order. A rearrangement of a bookshelf or a change in schedule may be unusually upsetting to a person with OCD.

Compulsions are irresistible urges to perform

actions which result from obsessive thoughts. For instance, a compulsive need to wash one's hands might result from an obsession with the avoidance of germs.

Compulsive activities are usually performed in a ritualistic fashion. Obsessive-compulsive individuals feel that they must touch things a certain number of times, check and recheck light switches and door locks, or take an exact number of steps between two points. The need to carry out these rituals tends to be driven by an overwhelming feeling that dire consequences will result if these behaviors are not executed correctly.

Studies indicate that about half of all Tourette syndrome patients demonstrate obsessive-compulsive thought patterns and behaviors. These tendencies often develop well after the onset of tics, and compulsions may consist of specific tics performed in mathematical sequence.[6]

Although OCD is often listed as a symptom of TS, many neurological researchers feel that the reverse is true, placing Tourette syndrome under the umbrella of obsessive-compulsive disorder. Several studies refer to TS as a tic-related form of OCD, but the nature of compulsions varies. Tourette patients are generally compelled to touch objects or people, whereas OCD sufferers without TS tend to be driven by fears, and feel they must perform rituals aimed at alleviating these fears.7

In addition to ADHD and OCD, Tourette syndrome researchers have drawn links to numerous other disorders. These problems may be symptoms, or simply parallel conditions, possibly stemming from some of the same neurochemical disturbances. Regardless, they occur more often in Tourette patients than in the population as a whole. The list includes depression, phobias, panic attacks, dyslexia and other learning disabilities, aggressive or oppositional behavior, stuttering, and sleeping problems. Researchers have also suggested links to eating disorders and addictive tendencies, but these connections are somewhat controversial.8

Tics: The Definitive Symptom of TS

Athough TS involves a variety of symptoms, motor and vocal tics continue to be the essential element in the diagnosis of this disorder. Tics can be broken down according to type and complexity.

Motor tics are involuntary, stereotyped movements of an appendage, muscle group, or body part. These are usually rapid, abrupt gestures, such as jerking the head, slapping the side, contorting the face, or twisting the torso. They can be performed singularly or in sequence.

Vocal (phonic) tics include snorting, clearing the throat, sniffing, or in more severe cases, making animal-like noises, screaming, or blurting out phrases.

Both motor and vocal tics are divided into two classes, *simple* and *complex*. *Simple tics* usually involve only one muscle group or body part, and have a very short duration. Stomping the foot is an example of a *simple motor tic*. A *simple vocal tic* is a brief noise made with the mouth, nose, or throat. Sniffs, grunts, throat clearing, clicking noises, or coughs are examples of simple vocal tics.

Complex motor tics consist of a combination of movements or gestures. They may be driven by obsessive urges, and involve several muscle groups. Examples include retracing steps, jumping over cracks in the sidewalk, or repeatedly opening and closing a door.

Unusual complex motor tics include *copropraxia* (the making of obscene or offensive gestures) and *echopraxia,* also called *echokinesis* (the repeating or mimicking of others' movements). *Coprographia* is the writing of obscene words or statements. These unusual motor tics tend to appear only in the more severe cases of TS.

A different type of complex motor tic, the *dystonic tic,* involves a slower movement or sustained action. A person may tightly grip an object for several seconds, hold a pose for an extended time, or tightly clench the teeth.

Complex vocal tics consist of repeated words, phrases, or noises. They often appear to be random or meaningless in nature, or they may fall into one of the following categories:

Echolalia is the repeating of others' sounds, words, or phrases in an echoing fashion. A person with TS may pluck a random phrase from a conversation and rehearse it until the original speaker's inflections are perfected, eventually developing an uncanny ability to imitate others. Often mistaken for intentional mockery, this involuntary mimicry can be maddening for friends or family members.

Palilalia is the repeating of one's own words or phrases. Upon completing a sentence, a person repeats a word or phrase from that sentence several times, with inflection, until the tic has run its course.

Coprolalia is a vulgar or offensive vocal outburst. It ranges from the quiet utterance of a profane word to the shouting of offensive or obscene sentences. Sometimes an objectionable word or phrase is blurted out in mid-sentence, entirely out of context. At other times, an obscene remark may erupt from complete silence, for no apparent, rational reason.[9]

Though not necessarily vulgar, coprolalia is by nature offensive. This embarrassing tic may also include the use of racist, sexist, or religious slurs, making it perhaps the most difficult social challenge facing the Tourette patient. It is not easy to hide or disguise, and is guaranteed to attract negative attention.

Because of its outrageous nature, coprolalia has received more press coverage than all other Tourette symptoms combined—yet it exists in less than 30 percent of TS cases. This emphasis on the sensational has caused both the medical community and the public to incorrectly assume that coprolalia is an essential symptom of TS. It is highly probable that many cases of Tourette syndrome are overlooked because the symptoms do not include uncontrollable bursts of profanity.

Another type of tic which is rarely discussed in Tourette literature is the *mental tic,* which involves no movement or vocalization, yet stems from an obsessive thought and the need to resolve that thought. It may consist of an unpleasant idea and an immediate urge to counter that idea with a mental ritual, such as repeatedly counting to ten. Mental tics often involve mathematical processes and a fascination with symmetry.

Mental coprolalia is like vocal coprolalia, except no sound is made. Instead, a profane thought pops in and out of the mind.

Sensory tics have both mental and physical elements, and consist of an uncomfortable sensation which may precede a motor or vocal tic, often related to a certain body part. For example, the mind may detect a build-up of energy or tension in a hand or foot.

The *phantom fixation* includes both mental preoccupation and motor activity. A person may sense an imaginary object and reach out to feel or move it, much like a mime touching an invisible wall. Although the symptom may appear to observers to be triggered by a series of hallucinations, it is not. This action is driven by a vague, yet convincing awareness that the phantom is there.[10]

Evaluation of Tourette Syndrome

A physician seeing a potential Tourette patient for the first time is faced with a challenge. There is no simple test for the detection of Tourette syndrome. In most cases, careful, repeated observation and questioning are the only diagnostic procedures.

Under certain circumstances, the patient may be able to repress symptoms for brief periods of time. However, when the urge becomes unbearable or the environment is more relaxed, the tics will emerge, frequently in an explosive manner. For this reason, the doctor may have to examine the patient several times. Candid video recordings are useful diagnostic aids, as they enable doctors to witness behaviors which patients may have concealed during an office visit.

Occasionally, a physician may order an *electroencephalogram* (EEG). This examination of electrical impulses in the brain has indicated abnormal activity in some TS patients. Another test, called *positron emission tomography* (PET scan), creates a visual image of the brain. Used more for research than diagnosis, this test has also shown unusual activity in some individuals with TS. Neither PET scan nor EEG results provide conclusive evidence of the disorder.[11]

Tourette syndrome is considered to be incurable, yet treatable. The severity of symptoms may be affected by physical or mental stress, the presence of another illness, or any number of other factors.

Mild cases do not require treatment as long as the patient is able to function well with no medication or therapy. Unless properly treated, more severe cases can destroy a person's quality of life. As understanding broadens, perhaps earlier diagnosis, more effective treatment, and ultimately a cure are on the horizon for all who are touched by this multifaceted and complex disorder.

Chapter four
A Tourette Story

Everyone who has experienced Tourette syndrome has a different story to tell. Tics and obsessions vary tremendously. Individual reactions to them vary as well. Yet there are basic experiences which many of us with TS tend to have in common. All too often, these include an unfortunate series of misunderstandings and fiascoes in the early stages of diagnosis and treatment.

Over a period of twenty years, I was tested and treated for everything from eye problems to manic depression. The possibility of Tourette syndrome was never mentioned; the cause of my odd behavior remained a mystery. Perhaps by telling my story, I can help others avoid the frustration of a similar ordeal.

As a child, I had boundless energy. I loved to run,

climb, and stay constantly busy. Although this is normal childhood behavior, I was more than just a busy kid. My activity level was excessive. I was constantly fidgeting, jerking, and squirming, especially when eating or trying to relax. My parents became concerned and had me examined by a number of physicians. The diagnosis was always the same: "He's just hyperactive. Eventually, he'll grow out of it."

As the years went by, it became apparent that this hyperactivity was something more than a temporary childhood ailment. It was a preface to a much more complex problem.

By the time I was twelve, my nervous energy had started to evolve—it seemed to be taking on a life of its own. Rather than disappear, my movements became more exaggerated.

My first real tics appeared in my early teens. I began to blink my eyes rapidly and repeatedly, and started jerking my arm up and down by my side. By the time I was a sophomore, these movements were occurring everyday, and continued to increase in both frequency and complexity throughout my high school years.

As I developed, so did the tics. The blinking and arm jerks would dominate for a while, and then a new set of gestures would take over, followed by another. I started jerking my head to the side, and at times would touch my nose repeatedly. Periodically, the old tics would return and combine with new ones, creating a virtual repertoire of unusual movements. Over the years, I learned to disguise a few, but was never able to hide them all. I had no idea why I moved this way, only that I could not stop.

As a result of the tics, I began to develop problems in school, both socially and academically. Due to the twitching of my hands and arms, my handwriting was poor and erratic, often bringing complaints from teachers. I began to feel inferior, and grew somewhat shy and reclusive because of my strange fidgeting. The constant struggle to conceal my symptoms was becoming more difficult. It was embarrassing and frustrating to have so little control over my body.

Still, I was lucky compared to most children with TS, because my symptoms remained relatively minor until my late high school years. By this time, I had already established friendships, and most of my classmates seemed to accept my odd nervous habits.

I was also fortunate with regard to vocal tics. The only ones I remember were an occasional clearing of the throat, snort, or grunt. I eventually learned to disguise most of them as allergy problems.

During this same period, obsessive-compulsive

rituals also began to develop. I recall counting the cracks in the school lunchroom ceiling tiles. At first, this felt like nothing more than a harmless game to occupy the time, but over the course of a few months, it grew increasingly necessary to count those cracks. Obsessions of this nature became more intense around my senior year of high school. I was rapidly becoming a slave to meaningless mathematical rituals.

The symptoms grew worse as I entered my early twenties. I quickly became out of control. The struggle against tics and obsessive-compulsive rituals took every ounce of my time and energy. Fighting this battle became the sole purpose for my existence. At this point, I began an exhaustive search for answers.

Through it all, my parents did everything they could to find the proper help for my condition—help which was then relatively unavailable. They were always supportive, and I often felt guilty for causing them to worry. I was totally baffled as to why I acted so strangely. I knew about hyperactivity, but had never heard that it could cause such bizarre symptoms. There had to be some other explanation.

By the time I reached my mid-twenties, I had been examined by several doctors, and had been given a number of medications for a variety of possible disorders. I had been addicted to (and had withdrawn from) a couple of different tranquilizers, and had also been prescribed some powerful sedatives, as a restful night's sleep had become a rare luxury. Still, the tics continued, so my family doctor advised me to seek psychotherapy.

My first psychologist thought that he could cure me through hypnosis, but the therapy proved to be unsuccessful. I was never able to relax enough to allow myself to be hypnotized. We had several long sessions, and he concluded that my twitches, jerks, and grunts were a physical manifestation of a deep psychological problem. After a few months, he diagnosed my condition as manic-depressive illness, and recommended several methods of treatment.

I followed the psychologist's instructions for improving my condition, but nothing seemed to work. At his recommendation, I remained on tranquilizers and learned some relaxation techniques. I also read the self-help books he suggested.

Even with this combination of therapy and medication, I continued to fidget, jerk my arms and legs, and clear my throat continuously. Eventually, I began to doubt the psychologist's assumption that manic-depressive illness was the true source of my problems. I decided to go back to a general practitioner, searching elsewhere for the elusive cause of my strange behavior.

My next doctor insisted that I was hyperactive and should try a stimulant. He explained that stimulants had worked well in hyperactive children, and might be able to help a twenty-seven year-old. Although he said that this was an experimental treatment for someone my age, I was ready to try anything. He instructed me to immediately stop taking my tranquilizer (I had been on the same one for a year and a half by now), and prescribed a drug called *Ritalin* instead.

For the next two weeks I was in a daze. I could not eat or sleep, and went through a rough withdrawal from the tranquilizer, suffering from vomiting, headaches, confusion, and extreme depression. The jerking symptoms became unbearable.

I finally had to stop the stimulant experiment, for fear that it was beginning to cause serious harm. I began to feel as if I had reached an all-time low. No one could figure out what was wrong with me, and every treatment I tried seemed to make things worse. As I became more and more depressed, this doctor, having exhausted his repertoire of therapy options, recommended a psychiatrist. Once again, I had come full circle.

Although attempts at psychotherapy had failed in the past, I followed up on the suggestion and had several sessions with a psychiatrist, hoping that his extensive training could help find some answers. After questioning me, he concluded that I suffered from self-induced stress, which caused the tics and obsessions. He also thought that my excessive blinking resulted from eye problems, and he referred me to an ophthalmologist.

The eye doctor prescribed some drops to help reduce dryness, but found no major problems. I tried the drops for months, but they proved to be of no avail.

During the months of therapy, the psychiatrist taught me a few techniques for breaking self-destructive mental habits. He continued to insist that excessive worry, overconcern, and a tendency to focus on the negative were the roots of my problem. His methods helped my attitude, but did nothing for my tics, so I moved on.

The guesswork continued for years. I was referred to specialist after specialist. The doctors checked for thyroid disorders, diabetes, and numerous other diseases.

Perhaps the absence of profane outbursts prevented anyone from considering TS as my problem. After all, virtually every report published at that time focused on one Tourettic symptom, coprolalia. In retrospect, I can only speculate.

With each failed diagnostic attempt, I became more discouraged. It is ironic that during this long period of trial and error, I probably did develop a few psychological problems. The long and unsuccessful search for the elusive skeleton in my mind's closet may have actually created one. I knew that something was very wrong, and that its origin was likely to remain a mystery forever. This knowledge was an unyielding burden to my mind.

I was finally diagnosed with Tourette syndrome at age thirty-two. Although I was not particularly pleased to have a strange neurological disorder, at least I had come to know the identity of my enemy, and this was a great relief.

Although it appeared that the battle was almost over, I soon realized that the struggle had just begun. It took years to discover the right combination of drugs for managing my tics and obsessions, and some of the prescribed medications created severe side effects, rendering me unable to function in everyday life.

Since that time, I have researched TS extensively in an effort to understand and cope with my condition. The sensations and emotions associated with it are interesting, varied, and complex. Words alone cannot adequately convey the mental activities endured with this disorder, for printed and spoken dialogue are limited forms of human communication. Although Tourette syndrome originates in the human brain, it embodies, and more importantly, embraces that which is inhuman.

Chapter five
An Interruption of Regular Programming

A person with Tourette syndrome must live two
lives, one dealing with the everyday stresses of health,
career, relationships, and finances—the other, a life of
struggle, an existence dedicated entirely to battling an
invisible enemy. While one portion of the mind main-
tains contact with the outside world, another is
engaged in intense combat with invading Tourettic
forces, fighting for the control of conscious thoughts
and actions.

Using an arsenal of ammunition, the foe attacks.
One of its most effective weapons is the obsessive
thought. An overwhelming notion is introduced which
interrupts concentration, breaks down the rational
mind's defenses, and allows this intruder to quickly
establish a state of mental mutiny. Its prey becomes

oddly convinced that a ritualistic sequence of tics must be carried out immediately. Within a fraction of a second, the initial obsession is followed by the enemy's second line of attack, an intense physical urge to tic.

In order to understand this combination of sensations, imagine you have a horrible itch which is driving you crazy. You must scratch it immediately and repeatedly until it can no longer be felt. Until it is scratched sufficiently, you are overpowered by a feeling that disaster will surely come. The nature of the disaster is not always clear, but the feeling of impending doom is without question.

When the consequences are known, they frequently involve your worst fears. The enemy may convince you that you will die, your house will burn, or a loved one's plane will crash if you fail to follow orders.

Whether vague or specific, the fear is just as real and overwhelming as anything in the universe, but it creates no actual terror or panic. These sensations are not perceived as immediate threats, but rather omens, urgent needs to take preventative measures. The rational, analytical mind is fully aware that there is no logical connection between moving a body part and preventing a disaster, yet it is convinced that there may be a connection, one which was somehow overlooked.

It is therefore an absolute necessity to tic and continue ticcing until the tension relaxes and the sense of premonition dissipates.

An excellent description of this phenomenon can be found in the Hope Press book, *Don't Think About Monkeys*. The following excerpt, reprinted with permission, dramatically relates the experiences of the father in a family of Tourette sufferers:

> *It is like a dark, murky night that never ends; relief is brief and superficial, and then abruptly consumed. There is a sense of hopelessness that what his body feels is constant. The sensations are real, sometimes obscure, often frightening, never absent.*
>
> *His body experiences a continuing series of peaks and valleys, but where, in other circumstances, the peak may mean elation or ecstasy and the valley tranquility, for the father the peak brings strain, confusion and pain, a sense than an unseen, unknown and unwelcome pressure is poking, pushing and shoving every part of his body.*
>
> *It is closing doors time and time again until sensations inside him announce, "It is okay now, the door is closed correctly," even though he knew it was closed correctly the first, second, third time and every*

time after that. It was closed correctly even when the muscles in his hand and wrist contort in pain from grasping the door handle so many times until it is the "correct" time.

It is rolling up the car window a dozen times, locking doors over and over again, wringing out wet rags to the point where every muscle and bone in his hand aches. It is turning lights on and off dozens of times until he has halved the life expectancy of the bulb.

It is reading a sentence in a book or in a newspaper four, five, six or so many times that he has memorized it. But it must be done correctly, eyes beginning on the first letter of the first word, including every letter of every word as the eyes move from left to right to the next line and finally to the punctuation mark. "No, dammit, it's not right, do it again!" his body screams. Then he quickly glances at the flashing lights on the clock that tick away the seconds, adding another dimension to the compulsive ritual. A dimension unrequested, yet quick to volunteer, that coerces him into letting it be part of his body, to join the "fun". Then he reads the line again. It is still not right. His eyes jump to the clock. He is prohibited from seeing the actual flash but must focus on the clock between flashes. Then he returns to the page for round five of this sparring match with clock and book.

It is touching an object with his right hand and then forced by an eerie feeling of duress to touch the same object with his left hand, then repeating that ritual time after time until his body tells him, "That's enough, I'm satisfied." He walks away, his energy and self-confidence diminished, then suddenly realizes that his body was only teasing him. It really was not satisfied. He returns to the same object and touches it again and again, first with the left hand, then with the right, or maybe twice with the left and twice with the right, or maybe...

Or perhaps his left hand does not wish to participate and he touches, touches with his right hand, unable to exhale until the need is satisfied. This time the body is not teasing, only temporarily inactive, a rest period that lasts for so little time. He walks away mumbling to himself, "Damn, why do I do it? Why can't I stop?"[12]

These nonsensical thoughts and urges are difficult to understand, because tics, obsessions, and their related mental activities are from a source other than the everyday, rational mind. Although tics seem to be senseless on the surface, they may make perfect sense and serve a well-calculated purpose to the Tourettic part of the brain.

It is as if the symptom-generating mind and the conscious mind operate independently, yet simultaneously. Each has its own agenda. The intellect can generally maintain control, but irrational obsessions will jump in at every opportunity, taking over until the tic is performed and the urge resolved.

With complex, repetitive, or ritualistic tics, the process of resolution can last for several minutes. A person may repeat a tic, much like a phonograph needle hanging up on a scratched record. In contrast, with simple tics, the sensation, tic, and subsequent feeling of relief can all take place in a fraction of a second.

A tic or ritual may also consist of not moving, rather than moving. A person may feel the need to "lock in" on an object and stare at it until the eyes actually begin to lose focus, unable to move until the brain sends the command that it feels satisfied.

The relentless attack of these tics soon becomes exhausting and frustrating. The feeling that some unwanted outside power is possessing the mind and body is highly irritating.

This takeover occurs much like a C.B. radio signal interrupting a radio or television broadcast. A radio tuned to a strong station is less likely to pick up interference than one which is tuned to a weaker signal. Likewise, when a person is extremely focused in work or play, the interference of tics and obsessions breaks in less often and with less intensity. There is no need to fight the urge to tic, as it is temporarily absent.

The mind's ability to squelch unwanted signals is virtually impossible to consciously achieve. It just happens. The relief is only temporary—it is inevitable that TS will break in with its relentless "interruption of regular programming."

I once had a job repairing copiers. Much of this work was fairly routine, and I could perform it with little concentration. Therefore, it was extremely difficult to do my job efficiently due to the incessant, overriding signals of TS and the resulting motor tics. Periodically, my focus would keep them locked out, but most of the time I was under "tic attack."

One day my tics were particularly bad and someone asked if I was being shocked by the machine. At the time, I was not in the mood for lengthy explanations, so I replied, "Just a little jolt, not too bad."

The tics sometimes caused me to break parts of the machine or bang my hands against sharp objects, creating aggravating small injuries. One symptom in particular appeared intermittently, severely interrupting the performance of my job. I would become unable to gently hold something in my hand, and unwillingly squeeze a part or tool with great pressure. This resulted in my breaking an expensive circuit board on one machine. I finally decided to quit the copier repair business, and focus fully on my primary occupation, playing music.

While it may seem strange that a person with such a potentially embarrassing illness would choose to perform on stage in front of an audience, I have always been totally absorbed by music and determined that TS would not stop me from pursuing it as a career. I do feel that I would be a better musician were it not for the disorder, because the tics make quality practice difficult. During a performance, however, the intense amount of concentration required to play music before an audience helps prevent the takeover of symptoms.

I have heard that others with TS experience the same phenomenon while heavily involved in a task, particularly one they enjoy. Perhaps it is this relief which has inspired many to choose music, theater, or sports as a career. Because these occupations require focus during a competition or performance, they provide excellent opportunities to minimize tics.

There are times when a person with TS appears to be controlling tics even while not absorbed in a demanding activity. This is a different phenomenon than the remission of symptoms due to intense focus. It also goes beyond the ability to temporarily suppress tics, and is an actual escape from the grip of the disorder.

On these infrequent occasions, the disorder seems to step back into the shadows and is not felt at all. It is almost as if the illness temporarily disappears, or enters a state of consciousness similar to sleep.

To others, it may appear that the person with TS has finally achieved self-control. This is an erroneous conclusion. The peaceful episode is merely a cease-fire, a break in the battle, one which is just as mysterious to the patient as it is to the observer.

Under normal conditions, the simplest, most fundamental tasks are sometimes the hardest to carry out. They require little focus, and provide no buffer against the invasion of tics, giving the intruder carte blanche. Shifting gears in an automobile, shaving, and pouring a cup of coffee may seem like simple tasks, but they can become dangerous, near impossible feats for those with tics.

A chore that I particularly dread is tuning my guitar, even with the convenience of an electronic tuner. Like every other guitarist, I pick up the guitar, pluck the E string, and reach for the first tuning key. My hand jerks back as if it has touched a hot iron. It then violently pounds against my side, sometimes causing deep bruises. While ignoring the pain, I reach for the key again, managing to get near it this time. Suddenly, the guitar leaps several inches forward, then slams back into my lower stomach. I cringe for a moment, then continue.

Over the years, I have become well practiced at disregarding the physical pain inflicted by severe motor tics. Although I am fully aware of the discomfort, I am usually able to deny both the impact of, and the reaction to the injury.

To the invading enemy, this pain may be perceived as pleasurable—not in a sadistic way, but as ver-ification of a successful attack. It seems to believe that physical pain caused by a violent tic indicates a victory, a hit, a winning score.

Ignoring the pain is relatively easy, but completing

the desired task is extremely difficult. I can't keep my fingers on the instrument's tuning keys long enough to make the necessary adjustments. With each attempt, I struggle to execute fluid and purposeful movements, but my ability to do so is quickly overridden. I eventually tune each string with a slow series of jerky motions, sneaking in only a split second of adjustment at a time. Without tics, I could tune the guitar in about three minutes—with them, it may take fifteen. To the Tourettic mind, this contest is a cruel, humorous game. To me, it is but one episode in a series of stressful experiences, and another of many reasons to detest Tourette syndrome.

Imagine for a moment that Tourette syndrome is actually a form of demonic possession, as was once believed. People with TS often feel as if an unwanted entity lives inside the brain, has a personality of its own, and sets up shop in order to carry out its daily routine. This invader has needs, urges, feelings of satisfaction, a sense of purpose, clear awareness of task completion, and the will to take over. It knows what it wants and will not take "no" for an answer. It can compel a person to perform acts which would never be carried out otherwise. If one resists, even manages to fight off the urge for a period of time, the entity will eventually win and make its victim pay dearly for the delay. The punishment is usually a much more severe explosion of the withheld tics.

When the person becomes fatigued from sickness, stress, or some other cause, the entity seizes the opportunity and has a field day. The host's natural defenses are down, and the invader can launch an unopposed attack, causing symptoms to appear in a more frequent, extreme manner.

The Tourettic demon has a memory as well. It can store a multitude of tics and obsessions and recall them years later. Some will disappear for a period of time, only to reappear with a vengeance as if they had never left. Tics and rituals continue to be added to the repertoire as this pseudo-parasite feeds from the memories and emotions of its victim.

The invading entity also sees things differently than the host, and reacts accordingly. It will tap into the victim's knowledge of morals and etiquette, and act in direct opposition to what it knows is proper conduct. In those with coprolalia, the demon will blurt out something offensive in an effort to humiliate the host into further submission.

Although coprolalia literally means "feces language," vocal outbursts of this type do not necessarily involve profanity. In one reported case, a TS patient often blurted out the word "hijack" when seated on an airplane.[13] The demon observed the situation and knew exactly what to do in order to create the most havoc.

It may also harbor some jealousy of the host's ability to get along with other people. In an attempt to undermine this ability, it will conjure up a number of offensive behaviors aimed at sabotaging the host's relationships. The invader will try to repulse or aggravate others around its victim, in order to fight its battle from the outside as well as the inside.

The demon can even force its hostage into self-harming behavior. I once had a tic attack so severe that I cracked several ribs by hitting myself in the side. This was obviously not an intentional act. I simply could not control the demon.

In the movie version of *The Exorcist*, one of the most disturbing scenes portrayed the possessed child stabbing herself with a crucifix while shouting profanity. Although this was a fictional story, this scene could easily have been a depiction of a severe Tourettic episode.

It is known that William Blatty, author of *The Exorcist*, studied a 1949 occurrence involving a young boy who was considered by the Catholic Church to be an actual victim of demonic possession. The church performed three rituals of exorcism in an attempt to help the child, whose symptoms included involuntary profane outbursts, growling, and violent, grotesque movements.

The final exorcism was thought to be successful, yet the results of the church's follow-up examination are not well documented. Expert physicians later determined that the boy's unusual demeanor resulted from Tourette syndrome, and the alleged success of the exorcism was attributed to a spontaneous remission of tics, commonly found in TS. If such a mistake can occur in the mid-1900's, it is no wonder that witnesses in the distant past mistakenly viewed tics as manifestations of possession.

This illusion of being enslaved by demons actually helped lead to the discovery of Tourette syndrome. Dr. Gilles de la Tourette became interested in the numerous accounts of spiritual possession reported throughout Europe in the 1800's. He investigated several cases of demoniac behavior, and largely through these studies, identified the syndrome which bears his name today.[14]

I do not believe in possession by demons. Any

references to demonic powers in this book are used for descriptive purposes only. It is my opinion that all alleged cases of demonic possession, if properly investigated, would turn up absolutely no evidence of the supernatural. Instead, these so-called "demons" would prove to be merely symptoms of a neurological, psychological, or physical illness. Unbelievably, reports of this nature continue. Imaginations run wild, witnesses exaggerate actual occurrences, and religious dogma has a strong suggestive influence on those who search for demons.

There are countless ways in which TS asserts its destructive powers. Over the years I have spent hundreds of dollars on dental bills, due to excessive grinding of the teeth. Others with TS have reported similar experiences. This activity may go unnoticed until sufficient damage to the teeth and gums brings it to a dentist's attention. Although many people grind their teeth during sleep, the Tourette patient may also grind and clamp teeth tightly together throughout the day, compounding the problem. Often a dentist will recommend a mouthpiece called a "night guard," which reduces damage from this destructive tendency.

Self-injury from TS may be much more blatant.

People bruise and scratch themselves, chew their lips and tongues, and break bones in their hands and feet from tics. On rare occasions, extreme tics of the head cause retinal detachment, resulting in blindness.[15]

Patients may also experience self-destructive urges. These are quite different from accidental injuries resulting from tics. They involve an obsessive thought which forces the person to deliberately perform a dangerous or painful act, such as closing the eyes while driving, or touching a hot stove. In the case of the latter, the burning pain acts as closure to the urge-relief ritual.[16]

There has been some debate as to whether Tourette syndrome tics are actually voluntary or involuntary. They are generally considered to be involuntary acts, yet the possibility that tics are intentional executions of movement or sound has been discussed.

In 1980, the *Archives of General Psychiatry* published a paper which detailed the experiences of a Tourette syndrome patient who recorded his observations of the sensations before, during, and after a tic. This patient, Joseph Bliss, concluded that his motor and vocal tics were voluntary acts performed for the purpose of satisfying unfulfilled urges. He stated that tics appeared to be involuntary to most witnesses, but actually were not. To the Tourettic mind, these acts are intentional.[17]

Some observers also assume that Tourette syndrome is caused by the random misfiring of neurons in the brain, and consequent reaction of the muscles affected. Tics are not that simple. Unlike convulsions, twitches, or spasms, in which the conscious mind merely observes the discomfort or movement after the fact, tics are purposeful in design and definitely deliberate.

The discussion of voluntary versus involuntary tics should clarify some misconceptions about Tourette syndrome. I have often been asked, "Why does your arm move like that?" It is difficult to explain, but my arm does not simply move. A chain of command is executed throughout the body's neuromuscular system, and the arm is ordered to move. However, the commander is not me—at least not the me I recognize as a conscious person. The tic must be performed in the correct, intentional manner necessary to relieve the urge and satisfy the master, which in this case, is the Tourette demon.

TS is so powerful that it can almost completely take

control over the mind and body, in some cases forcing a person to withdraw from society. Severely affected patients may go for months without leaving home, due to embarrassment, shame, and public aversion to their strange behavior.

Generally, the only way doctors have been able to calm this demon is to drug it. Unfortunately, to drug the demon is also to drug the person in which it resides. The enemy can never be destroyed, because it is a part of the patient. It knows every thought that enters the mind and it cannot be tricked. These factors make it difficult to subdue the disorder without negatively affecting the conscious mind of the patient.

During a radio interview, I was asked to point out the differences between *Tourette syndrome* and *Multiple Personality Disorder (MPD),* a condition in which the patient displays two or more distinctly individual personalities. The reporter pointed out that both disorders seem to have the power to "possess" the sufferer. This observation is correct, but the two disorders are not related.

Tourette syndrome is an inherited condition, and its outward symptoms are induced by chemical imbalances in the brain. The primary psychological effects of TS are anxiety and depression which result from dealing with the biological disorder.

Multiple Personality Disorder is considered to be a psychologically-based condition in which the patient develops different personalities in order to cope with emotional trauma, such as abuse as a child. Because an enormously high percentage of MPD cases involve patients who have known histories of upsetting experiences, this rationale is thought to be accurate.

Another significant difference between the two disorders lies in the patient's awareness of inner conflict. A person with MPD may be unaware that other personalities occupy the same body. There is no rapid, relentless tug-of-war for control. Either one personality rules or another. MPD is a *disassociative* disorder in which a person loses association with his or her primary personality.

Tourette syndrome is different. The patient is totally aware that the mind is engaged in a never-ending struggle for control. The tics, obsessions, and compulsions may dominate briefly, but the person is always mindful of the situation and feels a dire need to recover command.

This awareness is both a blessing and a curse. It is a blessing in that a person with TS can usually gain control in a matter of seconds, before the intrusive entity continues its often reprehensible and destructive behavior. But it is a horrible experience to witness oneself uncontrollably performing contortions, vocalizations, and gestures, even for a moment, while being fully cognizant of their grotesque nature.

Chapter six
Causes of Tourette Syndrome

The human brain is an electrochemical mechanism. Its chemical make-up, operating in concert with electrical impulses, helps to form our personalities. A change in this chemistry can cause a change in behavior.

Imbalances within the brain are responsible for a myriad of neurological disorders, including Tourette syndrome. If a human can be regarded as an electro-chemical being, TS may be considered an entity of the same nature, only one born of malfunction.

There is little doubt that Tourette syndrome is genetic in origin. Researchers such as David E. Comings M.D., Director of the Tourette Syndrome Clinic and the Department of Medical Genetics at the City of Hope National Medical Center, have extensively studied the hereditary aspects of TS. Utilizing pedigree studies of the families of patients, he and other scientists have concluded that Tourette syndrome is an inherited disorder.

A few researchers question the certainty of this conclusion. In about one-fourth of Tourette patients investigated, pedigree studies indicate no apparent genetic explanation for the transference of the disorder. One school of thought suggests that these may be spontaneous cases related to injury or difficulties during birth.[18]

Most geneticists maintain, however, that the disorder is always inherited, despite the fact that it is sometimes difficult to find a relative with symptoms. Since the gene (or genes) responsible for TS is believed to also cause OCD, ADHD, sleeping problems, and other, more obscure conditions, its presence may not always be obvious. In some family members, it may not reveal itself at all, providing no clue of the existence of TS in the patient's ancestry.[19]

This gene, sometimes called the *Gts* (or Gilles de la Tourette syndrome) gene, primarily affects the functioning of *neurotransmitters*, the brain's chemical messengers, which carry signals from one *neuron* (nerve cell) to another across a gap called a *synapse*. The principal neurotransmitters thought to be involved are a group called *biogenic amines*, which include *serotonin, dopamine,* and *norepinephrine*.[20]

One important factor in Tourette syndrome's influence on behavior is its ability to cause a "disinhibiting" effect. When this disorder takes over, an individual performs acts or makes statements which would otherwise be censored by the conscious mind.

Serotonin is the neurotransmitter believed to be primarily responsible for censorship, or inhibition. Both human and animal studies have proven that an imbalance of this chemical can cause drastic behavioral changes, leading to aggression, obsessive-compulsive thinking, depression, addictive tendencies, and other conditions. The brain of a person with Tourette syndrome may not adequately process serotonin, resulting in rampant, ungoverned thought processes.

Dopamine, another neurotransmitter, affects muscle movement as well as behavior. A deficiency of dopamine has been found in patients suffering from *Parkinson's disease*, which is characterized by difficulty in movement execution, slow or rigid motion, and tremor. Increased dopamine levels can cause exaggerated behaviors, including aggression and increased sexual activity. Overactive dopamine-processing neurons, or excessive dopamine levels in certain parts of the brain, may also result in the rapid tic movements found in TS patients.

Dopamine processing is regulated by another neurotransmitter, *norepinephrine* (also called *noradrenalin*), which modulates the actions of many of the brain's chemicals. An imbalance of norepinephrine upsets overall neurochemical harmony, allowing the onset of depression, TS, and a number of other disorders.

Norephinephrine and dopamine work closely together to stimulate behavior, while serotonin inhibits behavior.[21] Too much of one, too little of another, or improper processing of any of these chemicals, can literally wreak havoc on a person's thoughts, emotions, and functions.

Hormones may also contribute to the chaos. Recent studies indicate a connection between excessive levels of the hormone *oxytocin* and obsessive-compulsive disorder, a close relative of Tourette syndrome. Although oxytocin's primary role is in childbirth and lactation, it also plays an important part in both grooming and social behavior. Increased levels of oxytocin have been found in many patients who regularly perform obsessive-compulsive cleaning or hygiene rituals.

Vasopressin, another hormone, regulates the intake and secretion of fluids in the body, and affects memory.

It has also been implicated in TS, although the nature and importance of its role, and the role of other hormones, is yet to be determined.[22]

Many of the chemical imbalances which cause tics and obsessions affect the structures of the brain known as the *basal ganglia*. These centers, located deep within the brain, act as relay stations for neurochemical messages.[23]

Imbalances can also affect the *limbic system*, the part of the brain which controls emotions. A disturbance within this system can cause decreased inhibitions and inappropriate reactions.

As many as seventy different chemicals in the brain may influence human behavior. The number contributing to TS is still unclear. The ongoing study of these substances will undoubtedly turn up additional clues for solving the complex riddle that is Tourette syndrome.

Chapter seven
The Drug Dilemma

Discovering the nature of a common illness and prescribing the appropriate medication is usually a relatively routine matter for a trained physician. Neurological disorders, however, can be much more difficult to properly diagnose and treat. The complexity of these disorders, the myriad of treatment options, and the potential adverse effects of medication must all be considered.

Before I was diagnosed with Tourette syndrome, I was prescribed a number of drugs which not only failed to help my symptoms, but caused annoying side effects. I soon grew tired of the headaches, confusion, exhaustion, blurred vision, and other problems associated with these drugs. Memories of those years now seem vague. Much was lost in the fog of inappropriate medication. I cannot remember some periods of my life, nor can I recall the name of every drug that I was prescribed. Many of these pharmaceuticals apparently acted as chemical sledgehammers, temporarily pounding every ounce of cognitive ability from my brain.

In spite of this, I was determined to cooperate with my doctors in an effort to find a solution to my mysterious problem. In retrospect, I realize that some of these physicians apparently had no clue as to what my illness could be, yet most seemed unwilling to admit it. They were merely shooting in the dark.

After being correctly diagnosed, I thought my years of living at the mercy of unpleasant side effects were over. I was wrong. It took six additional years of experimentation before my physicians and I were able to find a proper combination and dosage of medications, one which reduced the symptoms without destroying my ability to function.

I was prescribed a major tranquilizer, and tried various dosages of it for years. I assumed that it was the only drug available for the treatment of TS. When I mentioned problems with side effects to my neurologist, a change in dosage was the only suggested remedy. My intolerance for this drug, combined with my lack of knowledge, resulted in years of unnecessary anguish. Finally, I began to research the subject. I also changed physicians.

Once aware that other medications were available, I started working, with my new doctor's help, to find a suitable treatment. Although experimentation was sometimes rough, even the most intolerable of drugs provided some escape from the relentless attack of tics. By this time, I had learned to accept the side effects as simply part of the quest.

In some cases, particularly with children, Tourette syndrome patients seem to be medicated primarily for the benefit of those around them. Once a person's tics are brought under control, those nearby feel relieved by the peace and quiet, but the patient may be stuck in a private nightmare. The true challenge for the physician is not only to control the disorder, but to preserve or improve the patient's quality of life in the process.

For a person with TS, the first and most important step is to find a doctor who is either knowledgeable about the available treatment options, or is willing to thoroughly research the topic. Physicians with a clear understanding of TS are aware that treatment of this complex disorder requires considerable involvement on the part of the patient. No blanket approach will work. If one medication is intolerable and another exists, the patient should be informed.

The patient has equal responsibility in the process. Ineffective drug therapy is not always the doctor's fault. If a medication is causing unpleasant side effects or if it is failing to reduce symptoms, the patient must speak up. Without this dialogue, even the best of physicians cannot sufficiently treat the disorder.

It can be quite a challenge for any physician to manage just one complex illness, such as obsessive-compulsive disorder. Tourette syndrome is particularly difficult to treat. The presence of so many symptoms and related conditions can create a neurological Medusa. One drug may alleviate a certain symptom but leave the others untouched. In some cases it can even make them worse.

A patient can become frustrated and fail to give the doctor adequate time to complete a necessary medication trial. Some drugs take months to reach their full effectiveness. Instant relief without adverse side effects is extremely rare.

With or without treatment of any kind, this complex disorder tends to change in both severity and nature. Throughout the years its tendency to wax and wane has caused many a patient, physician, and psychologist to misjudge the effectiveness of various therapeutic methods.

Outside influences also have an enormous effect on TS. Pressure in the workplace, stress at home, or any uncomfortable situation may trigger an increase in both tics and obsessive-compulsive behaviors. Sleeping too much or too little, excitement, anticipation, and other emotional stimuli can drastically affect symptoms.

Any number of foods, drinks, and medications can have an effect on TS as well. Over-the-counter cold remedies and caffeine are good examples. These substances can aggravate symptoms, which may lead to an incorrect evaluation of the patient's medication. Diet, drinking habits, and use of over-the-counter prepartions should be discussed with a physician in order to help minimize confusion.

There are no perfect treatments for Tourette syndrome, yet given the wide array of available options, most patients no longer have to accept the choice between an intolerable treatment and an intolerable disorder.

Chapter eight
Treatment of TS

Because TS results from imbalances of neurotransmitters and other chemicals in the brain, the
primary approach to controlling symptoms continues
to be the administration of drugs which affect these
neurochemicals. Various medications and techniques
are used to treat the disorder, and although personal
narrative appears in this discussion, in no way is the
author either recommending or condemning the use of
any specific treatment. Only a qualified physician can
safely recommend methods for the management of
Tourette syndrome.

Since 1961, the drug of choice for the treatment of
TS has been *Haldol* (haloperidol). Haldol belongs to the

group of medications known as *neuroleptics, anti-psychotics,* or *major tranquilizers.* It works by blocking dopamine receptors in the brain, and is successful in about 80 percent of all cases in relieving tics. Many patients, upon beginning therapy with Haldol, notice an immediate improvement in their symptoms.

Although this drug is successful in diminishing tics, it is not well tolerated by some patients. Haldol is a powerful medication used primarily in the treatment of psychological disturbances. It can produce unpleasant side effects such as cognitive blunting (decreased ability to learn), sedation, dysphoria (depression, irritability), weight gain, akathisia (restlessness), and nightmares.[23]

Symptoms similar to those found in Parkinson's disease may also result from the long-term use of neuroleptics. These include muscle rigidity, tremors, and *tardive dyskinesia,* a potentially irreversible condition characterized by various unusual movements, particularly chewing motions.[25] In order to minimize possible adverse effects while achieving the maximum benefits of neuroleptic drugs, the physician must carefully monitor the patient's response to treatment.

When I first went to a neurologist and received a diagnosis of Tourette syndrome, both the doctor's diagnostic manner and his way of prescribing medication struck me as peculiar. After diagnosing my problem, he brought an intern into the examining room.

"My new intern has never seen anyone with Tourette syndrome," he said. "Could you do a tic for him?"

I tried to describe my tics to the young doctor, but explained to both of them that I could not tic on command. It does not work that way. I felt that this was a very unusual request. Surely this experienced doctor knew that TS patients cannot voluntarily perform motor or vocal tics like a dog doing tricks.

After a brief reflex examination and a few more questions concerning my symptoms, I was prescribed Haldol in a rather loose fashion. I was told that I could alter the dosage to some degree, according to the severity of my symptoms. The doctor said that I might experience some side effects, and that I could lower the dosage if needed. It was basically a situation involving the lesser of two evils—the disorder versus the treatment.

After taking only a small dosage for a day or two, I became zombie-like, unable to think clearly. I could not perform any task which required concentration, and suffered from both fatigue and restlessness at the same time. Despite these problems, I continued with the medication for several months, determined to endure whatever was necessary in order to keep the tics at bay. The tics did diminish considerably, but at the cost of my ability to function. I remember looking at the clock one day. It was two o'clock. I could clearly read the time, but in my confused state I wondered, "What in the world does two o'clock mean?"

I eventually decided to try another neurologist. He confirmed the diagnosis of TS, but also preferred Haldol. He attempted to adjust my dosage, assuming that I might be taking too much. I tried the new dosage for almost two years, but continued to feel like a mindless automaton. By this time I had given up any kind of work which required serious concentration. I was in a constant state of confusion, unable to perform the simplest of tasks. I was also experiencing tremendous depression and a tendency to nod off to sleep while driving. I realized that I had to change my medication and find a doctor who would offer alternate therapies. Haldol wasn't the right drug for me.

Although my next physician agreed that neuroleptics were not a feasible treatment option in my case, these drugs are effective in the management of TS in many individuals. Other medications of this type include *Orap* (pimozide), *Prolixin* (fluphenazine), and *Risperdal* (risperidone). These compounds work in much the same way as Haldol, but seem to produce fewer side effects in some patients.[26]

Another drug used to treat Tourette syndrome is clonidine. The brand name of clonidine is *Catapres,* and it has been used as an antihypertensive (high blood pressure medication) for years. It has also proven to be effective in reducing TS symptoms in over half the patients who have tried it, particularly those with mild to moderate cases.

Symptom relief usually occurs more gradually than with neuroleptics, but the side effects are often much less bothersome. Clonidine's reported side effects include fatigue, racing thoughts, insomnia, low blood pressure, and headaches.[27]

Clonidine's role in treating TS centers around its effect on the neurotransmitter norepinephrine. The drug inhibits the production of norepinephrine in parts of the brain, which in turn alters serotonin and dopamine levels, and is usually administered in either pill form or as a skin patch. Many doctors prefer the skin patch because it allows the drug to be slowly absorbed, providing an even dosage throughout the day. Some patients must take the medication in pill form because of irritation from wearing the patch.

Due to potentially dangerous withdrawal symptoms, a patient cannot suddenly stop taking clonidine after prolonged use. Under the guidance of a physician, the dosage must slowly be reduced, usually over a period of weeks.[28]

Clonidine initially proved to be a godsend in my case. During my Haldol years, I had grown to believe that I was doomed to spend the rest of my life either as a drugged-out zombie or an untreatable sufferer of Tourette syndrome.

Finally, I was informed about an organization called *The Tourette Syndrome Association, Inc. (TSA)*. I contacted them for help. They sent a list of pamphlets and medical publications containing information about TS. I was relieved to find that many drugs were being used for the management of this disorder, not just neuroleptics.

After reading the literature I became interested in clonidine. The information included several interviews with patients who were taking the medication. Their accounts of clonidine's effectiveness in reducing tics were encouraging. Complaints of side effects were minimal.

I took the information to my family doctor, who was interested and supportive. He agreed that we should try clonidine. He carefully monitored my blood pressure as we gradually increased the dosage.

Within a few weeks my tic symptoms began to diminish. The drug also had a calming effect, reducing my tendency to become frustrated or angry. For the first time in my life I felt significant relief from TS symptoms, with no severe impairment of function.

I took clonidine for about six years, with considerable benefit and few side effects. The worst consequence was a feeling of fatigue, even when I was rested. Eventually, I noticed a reduction in the drug's benefit, but no decrease in the fatiguing side effects. My doctor suggested that I slowly reduce, and finally discontinue the drug. My tics increased, but my exhaustion evaporated. Only time will tell if I will continue to function well without the medication.

Like virtually all drugs, clonidine is not perfect. All things considered, it is one of the most well-tolerated and effective drugs used in the treatment of TS.

There are also numerous antidepressants which are useful in controlling the non-tic symptoms associated with Tourette syndrome. Patients with severe obsessive-compulsive symptoms, panic attacks, aggressive behavior symptoms, or depression may benefit tremendously from these medications. The use of antidepressants in the management of TS, OCD, and related disorders has increased dramatically in the past few years.

Due to the various physiological effects of antidepressants, extreme caution must be used if one type is discontinued and another started. For example, one family of antidepressants *(MAO inhibitors)* can clash with other drugs and certain foods, resulting in serious complications.[29] It is important to discuss the use of any previous medication with a doctor before changing drugs.

One major group of antidepressants is referred to as *serotonin re-uptake blockers, serotonin re-uptake inhibitors,* or *selective serotonin re-uptake inhibitors (SSRI's)*. These medications work by inhibiting the reabsorption of serotonin at the gap between neurons, the synapse. In addition to controlling depression, SSRI's are particularly beneficial in managing the symptoms of obsessive-compulsive disorder. Reported side effects include headache, lack of sexual desire, sexual dysfunction, insomnia, and loss of appetite.[30]

Luvox (fluvoxamine), *Zoloft* (sertraline), *Serzone* (nefazodone), and *Paxil* (paroxetine) are among the newest drugs in this class, but perhaps the best known of all serotonin re-uptake inhibitors is *Prozac* (fluoxetine). Every drug in the SSRI family is different, but each centers its effect on serotonin.

A relatively new drug, *Effexor* (venlafaxine), is both an SSRI and a norepinephrine re-uptake inhibitor. This drug is also proving to be useful in the treatment of depression and obsessive-compulsive disorder.

I have taken Prozac for several years and feel that it has been an effective tool in calming both my obsessive-compulsive and depressive symptoms. I also seem to cope with stress more effectively than I did before taking Prozac. This benefit can indirectly help control tics, because TS symptoms are often amplified by stress. I have suffered no major side effects from this drug.

Another group of antidepressants, known as *tricyclics,* is also used to treat TS. One of these drugs, *Anafranil* (clomipramine), has been used in Europe for years to control obsessive-compulsive symptoms, and is now being used in the U.S. as well.

Tofranil (imipramine) and *Norpramin* (desipramine) are also commonly used tricyclics. These drugs are particularly effective against symptoms of TS associated with attention deficit hyperactivity disorder. Because they are antidepressants, they also aid in controlling the depression often seen in TS patients.

Drugs in other categories, such as *Klonopin* (clonazepam), *Lithium* (lithium carbonate), *Valium* (diazepam), and *Inderal* (propranalol) have also been used successfully in the management of TS. Most drugs used to treat TS were originally developed and approved to treat other disorders and later found to be effective against tics and obsessions. The list of treatments for Tourette syndrome is growing every year, as more existing drugs prove to be beneficial, and new medications are discovered. Because individuals react so differently to drugs, months or years of trial and error may be necessary in order to find the best treatments for Tourette syndrome. No patient wants to be a guinea pig, but experimentation is sometimes unavoidable.

In the past few years a debate has continued among physicians over the use of stimulants to treat children with attention deficit hyperactivity disorder. Stimulants can have a calming effect in pediatric patients, but some researchers claim that they can trigger the onset of tics or even full-blown Tourette syndrome in certain people. Others argue that the hyperactive child who develops tics was destined to do so with or without the use of the stimulants.

Although ADHD is prevalent among TS patients, the reverse is not true. In hyperactive children who do not have TS, stimulant therapy can be extremely beneficial. Caution should be used in treating any patient with ADHD who exhibits tics, as most researchers agree that stimulant use may cause pre-existing tic symptoms to become worse.[31]

Because TS can cause socially unacceptable behavior, a patient may develop problems coping with the resulting rejection and embarrassment. Feelings of low self-esteem, guilt, anger, and frustration often accompany a disorder which places a person in an awkward position every day. The assumption that others are watching every move and making negative judgments, whether true or not, often creates emotional trauma. Psychotherapy can prove beneficial for patients experiencing these feelings.

Psychologists also offer methods for managing the primary symptoms of TS. These techniques (such as substituting an oncoming tic with a less obvious one) are extremely helpful in many cases. Breaking bad habits, reducing stress, challenging obsessive-compulsive urges, and developing relaxation techniques can all have therapeutic benefits. While psychotherapy alone is generally not successful in stopping tics, its use in conjunction with proper medication may prove to be the most effective method of treatment.

Family members of the patient may also benefit from counseling. Feelings of guilt, shame, and anger commonly affect those who must deal with the frustrations of raising (or growing up with) a Tourettic child. A qualified therapist may be able to help parents better understand and cope with the inner mental struggles their child must face daily.

Openly discussing personal experiences with

others affected by TS can also be helpful. The TSA and other organizations sponsor chapters in most major cities, many of which schedule regular support group meetings.

People with Tourette syndrome frequently face their most difficult times as school children. Behavioral therapy, combined with specialized educational techniques, can be of considerable help in dealing with the social and learning difficulties experienced by many Tourettic students. This is particularly true in children who also have attention deficit hyperactivity disorder.

Although traditional Western treatments are the most widely used in the U.S., there are alternatives available to the adventurous TS patient. Around the world, Chinese herbal medicine and homeopathic medicine are among the oldest and most widely practiced of the healing arts. Both of these disciplines operate on a different set of principles than those of conventional Western medicine. Concentration is focused less on quick cures for specific symptoms and more on the patient's overall health. Emphasis is placed on strengthening and balancing the vital forces within, allowing the body to heal itself.

Chinese herbal medicine refers to this vital essence as *qi* (pronounced "chee"). According to ancient philosophy, *qi* permeates the universe and enters the body through the intake of food, liquids, and air, directly affecting the state of a person's health. By achieving an internal balance between opposing forces of nature, known as *yin* and *yang*, and by acquiring proper communication within the body among the natural elements of fire, wood, water, earth, and metal, the patient attains a strong *qi,* resulting in emotional and physical well-being.

When this balance is upset, disease occurs. The goal of the herbalist is to encourage the *qi* to flow freely by correcting the sources of imbalance.

Proper balance is ideally achieved by lifestyle and diet. If needed, the herbalist may prepare a tea or potion comprised of various herbs, minerals, barks, berries, or powdered animal parts to aid in the healing process. Interestingly, several of these substances have found their way into the pharma-copoeia of conventional Western medicine. Although the philosophy of *qi* is far from the mainstream in Western cultures, patients with a variety of ailments have claimed to find relief in the steeped concoctions prescribed by their venerable Chinese herbalists.

After years of conventional treatment, I decided to give Eastern medicine a try. I was told of an herbal medical center in a large city nearby, so I made an appointment. The walls of the small office were lined with hundreds of jars labeled with Chinese characters, and filled with various substances ranging from whole strips of tree bark to insect parts. The herbalist, who spoke poor English, asked me to find the name of my disorder in a book and point it out to him. He then tapped his finger on my pulse, looked into my eyes, and examined my tongue. His diagnosis was that my earth and wood elements, representing specific organs and emotions, were not communicating properly. He prescribed a tea made from herbs, bark, and several indescribable components.

I drank the foul-tasting tea for a few weeks, noticing no relief from symptoms. At the time, my doctor had prescribed dosage changes in my regular medication as well, which may have diminished the herbal treatment's benefits. Someday I may attempt the herbal method again and stick with the regimen for several months. The original experiment was interesting, but inconclusive. For now, I continue to be in the caring hands, or as some might say, the ferocious grip of traditional Western medicine.

Homeopathy is an alternative medical practice which has also attracted Tourette patients. Dr. Manfred Mueller, D.H.M., D. Hom, C.C.H. (Doctor of Homeopathic Medicine, Diplomat in Homeopathic Medicine, Certified Classical Homeopath) of Durham, North

Carolina, claims to have achieved a success rate of 80 percent in curing children of all TS symptoms, although he admits that it may take months or years to exact a complete recovery. Improvement depends largely on the amount of medication which has been previously prescribed to the patient, the underlying predisposition of the patient, and the patient's willingness to persevere.

Dr. Mueller reemphasizes that homeopathy utilizes an entirely different set of principles than conventional medicine. Since each case is different, a doctor must first determine the source of an individual's disorder. According to Mueller, TS may be brought on by an interplay between an existing sensitivity (predisposition) and a trigger (environmental stimulus).

In order to pursue the homeopathic approach, the patient must first discontinue the use of all other medications. Initial treatment is for the residual effects of these drugs, which employ a suppressive method of action. For this reason, it is more difficult, but certainly not impossible, to treat adults, many of whom have been prescribed suppressive drugs for years.

Dr. Mueller explains that in order to ease the transition into the new treatment, the patient may be given a temporary palliative homeopathic or herbal medication. Homeopathic treatment is a one on one, closely supervised process, especially during this difficult withdrawal period. It should never be attempted without the strict supervision of a physician trained in the field.

The next step is to treat for the presumed triggering cause of the disorder. A careful case history must be taken, as these triggers may include immunizations, past medication for various problems, and environmental factors. Only after eliminating all acquired iatrogenic and environmental causes can one move to the final stage of treatment, in which the underlying condition, the predisposition which made the patient vulnerable to begin with, is addressed.

Medicines are selected on an individual basis for each patient, as no two cases are the same. Homeopathic medicines are sold in accordance with a separate pharmacopoeia, which is FDA approved. The medicines evoke a curative response which allows the body to gradually heal the condition. They are harmless and free from adverse side effects.

Alternative disciplines for the management of TS also include nutrient therapies and the avoidance of allergens. Nutrients recommended for TS patients are believed to improve overall brain function, increase oxygenation of brain tissues, and help rid the brain cells and bloodstream of *lipopfuscin,* an unwanted by-product of fats and unattached oxygen molecules, known as free radicals. These nutrients are also believed to affect the balance of neurotransmitters within the brain. Among them are choline, lecithin, and vitamins A, B, and E. Whole grain foods, legumes, nuts, and fish are rich in these and other potentially helpful substances. Trained nutritionists are able to determine the types and quantities of foods and supplements needed to achieve a proper balance.

Researchers have found that allergic reactions to certain foods and irritants may also increase tics. Alteration of diet, lifestyle changes, and a regimen of fasting may lessen these negative responses.

Many forms of alternative medicine exist, and some may ultimately prove superior to conventional treatments. Unfortunately, a current lack of scientific data prevents researchers from adequately documenting the effectiveness of alternative therapies.[33] Perhaps in the future, this informational void will be filled.

Chapter nine
The Less Obvious Symptoms of TS

The list of potential Tourette symptoms only begins with tics, obsessions, and compulsions. Debate continues over whether certain related conditions are actual symptoms of Tourette syndrome or independent problems, which happen to crop up more often in TS patients. Although many of these occur in people who do not have the disorder, the abnormally high percentage of Tourette patients who experience them indicates that there is a genetic and chemical link, and that they are in all likelihood symptoms. Additional data must be studied before researchers can reach an overall agreement. For the sake of discussion, I refer to these conditions as "less obvious symptoms of TS," which seems to be the generally accepted consensus.

Phobias are irrational fears of specific objects, people, animals, places, or activities. People in all walks of life experience phobias, and for some, they can be debilitating.

On the surface, a tendency toward social phobias seems inevitable for people with TS. Years of embarrassing tics and awkward behavior can cause anyone to feel uneasy in social situations. This rational uneasiness can become obsessive, developing into a full-blown phobia, such as *ochlophobia* (fear of crowds), *xenophobia* (fear of strangers), or *anthrophobia* (fear of people). Studies indicate that Tourette patients may also inherit the tendency to develop multiple phobias which have nothing to do with being in public. The fear of being alone and the fear of water are examples.

I have always had a strange fear of accidentally writing incorrect letters or inappropriate words. Although I have never experienced either coprolalia or coprographia, given the nature of Tourette syndrome, I suppose this fear is only natural. Consequently, I rarely write letters by hand, relying on a word processor instead. This allows me to check and recheck my work before it is printed for others to see. I am not sure if this nagging fear is a phobia or an obsessive-compulsive behavior, but it drives me to repeatedly examine checks or letters for potentially embarrassing mistakes.

TS is not a mental illness, but sometimes it mimics one. Symptoms which resemble those of *autism* may occur in TS patients, including restricted interests, poor social interaction, and inferior communication abilities.

There are indications that autism may actually be linked to the gene (or genes) responsible for Tourette syndrome. This does not imply that those with TS have a higher incidence of autism, only that they must sometimes endure similar symptoms, and that perhaps these symptoms originate from the same source. Interestingly enough, many of these autistic symptoms are also associated with OCD and ADHD, whose close relationships to TS are well known.

Sleep problems, including difficulty falling asleep, restless sleep, and early awakening, are reported in many TS cases. These may result from sensations of increased internal energy and inability to relax, both mentally and physically. Other problems, including sleepwalking and bed-wetting are also common.

There has been considerable debate concerning the relationship between nocturnal motor activities and TS. Early reports stated that tics completely disappear during sleep, but later studies indicate that they continue throughout the night in some patients.[34] Because of the known relationship between Tourette syndrome and hyperactivity, excessive movements during sleep may also appear which are not true tics.

I do not believe that I have had a solid night's sleep in twenty years. The mental activities of Tourette syndrome seem to jump into overdrive as soon as I try to relax, and I become plagued with obsessive thought patterns and tics. Some mornings my only indication of having slept at all is my recollection of a dream. Much like tics, these sleep problems increase and decrease with time. Periodically I have taken pre-scribed sleeping pills, but I avoid their long-term use, as many are addictive.

Panic attacks are sudden feelings of overwhelming fear, apprehension, terror, or doom, usually brought on with little or no provocation. Many panic attack sufferers experience rapid heartbeat, sweating, short-ness of breath, and dizziness. These periods of intense anxiety occur in about one-fourth of all TS patients, and can be extremely upsetting or completely in-capacitating.

Those with TS are also at risk for *depression* from both genetic and environmental sources. Commonly, depression develops because of low self-esteem, rejection, and embarrassment brought on by tics.

Studies indicate that with or without the distress of tics, Tourette patients may carry genes which make them prone to bouts of depression, including the extreme mood swings associated with *bipolar (manic-depressive) disorder*.

The excessive drinking of fluids is called *polydipsia*. This symptom is believed to be linked to abnormal levels of the hormone vasopressin, which helps to regulate water processing in the body. Some cases of polydipsia may result from obsessive-compulsive urges, in which the TS patient is driven by an obsession with fluid intake.

People with TS sometimes complain of *heat intolerance* (discomfort when in warm surroundings). They feel hot, even when their environment is cool. The exact mechanism behind this symptom is unknown, although it is possibly hormonal in origin.

I never wear sweaters, and rarely wear a coat, unless it is extremely cold. I have often felt panicky, as if unable to breathe, when in warm environments. One side effect of the drug clonidine is its tendency to make one feel cooler, which has been beneficial in helping to relieve my heat intolerance.

It is common for people with TS to have an *intolerance to stress*. This symptom can be especially upsetting on several levels. Not only does stress increase the severity of tic symptoms, it causes a feeling of exhaustion. Most people feel drained when under stress, but TS patients tend to suffer fatigue to an inordinate degree.

A cycle of stress seems to form in which the cause and effect can become hard to discern. A chicken and egg scenario develops—do the symptoms cause stress, or does stress cause the symptoms?

The act of ticcing alone may be the initial cause. Excessive internal energy, difficulty focusing thoughts, and obsessive-compulsive behavior can add to the burden. The internal battle against these symptoms is, in itself, a major stressor.

Additional stress may result from the embarrassment of tics. The curious stares and expressions of disapproval can make a person with TS feel uncomfortable in social situations. Ironically, this can lead to exaggerated ticcing, and consequently more social discomfort, as the stress cycle worsens.

Conditions at work or at home may contribute heavily to an increase in stress, aggravating tics and exhaustion. The fatiguing side effects of medication make the load even heavier to carry.

Dyslexia is the inability to read words properly. People with dyslexia often reverse letters when writing, or omit words while reading. This condition is one of many learning disabilities found in TS patients. Others include difficulty paying attention, impatience, inability to listen, and excessive talking—symptoms commonly associated with ADHD.

Loss of fine-motor coordination can occur in varying degrees. This loss may contribute to poor handwriting skills, and can make it difficult to perform a variety of intricate manual operations.

In some cases, *migraine headaches* are thought to be genetically related to Tourette syndrome. Improper serotonin metabolism is instrumental in both migraines and TS, providing evidence of a genetic connection between the two.

Poor memory, a known symptom of ADD, may also present a problem for TS patients. Memory loss can appear as either a side effect of medication, or as a direct result of the disorder.

Racing thoughts can add to the learning and sleeping problems of TS patients. These thoughts, which rapidly appear and disappear, can lead to feelings of confusion. Like poor memory and insomnia, racing thoughts may also be caused by medication.

A number of other less-discussed conditions can occur in Tourette patients. Due to a lack of controlled studies, the percentage of cases in which they exist is not known. These include impulsive behavior, rapid mood swings, irritability, oppositional behavior, speech problems, cravings for sugar, and inappropriate sexual behaviors.[35] Each case is unique, and these conditions may exist in an individual in varying degrees, or not at all.

Chapter ten
Dealing With Society

I was sitting in a restaurant trying to eat a sandwich when a young man approached and began rapidly asking questions: "Hey man, what are you on? What drug are you coming down from? Do you need help? Are you sure you're okay?"

I thanked him for his concern and assured him that I was not suffering from drug withdrawal and did not need help. He assumed, as have many others, that a person jerking about and shaking must be having a reaction to a street drug, such as cocaine or heroin.

My odd table manners often seem to fuel this suspicion. Due to tics, I constantly spill things or shake the food off my fork. In order to avoid embarrassment when eating out, I frequently try to find a hiding place, such as a seat located in the rear of the restaurant. It is difficult enough to control tics while eating at home—I do not need the added stress of an audience.

Sometimes circumstances make it impossible to escape from people, their curious stares and inappropriate reactions. A few years ago, I was singing a vocal track in a recording studio. Much to my surprise and embarrassment, the engineer recorded my grunting between verses, then played it back to the musicians in the control room. I had been wearing headphones during the recording process and had no idea that I was having vocal tics. Everyone in the control room thought that this joke was funny, but I found it to be tasteless and irritating. It was difficult for me to control my temper, but I finally managed to laugh it off.

Public displays of Tourettic behavior can sometimes lead to more serious problems. In my college years, I was quietly walking across a campus parking lot on my way to class. The police pulled up and said they wanted to speak with me. They asked several questions about what I was doing, where I had been, and where I was going. The officers commented that I appeared to be extremely nervous, and questioned the reasons for my jerky movements. At the time I did not yet know the cause of my fidgeting, and was unable to give them a satisfactory answer. After a few minutes they evidently decided that I was harmless, thanked me for my cooperation, and moved on.

Understandably, it was upsetting that the police singled me out of thousands of college students for questioning. I assume that they saw me ticcing and thought that I might be either dangerously crazy or on drugs.

Fortunately, the only consequence of this particular encounter was that I was late for class. I have heard of others with TS who were actually held in custody by the police until the misunderstanding was cleared up.

People generally feel either aversion or sympathy for a person with tics. The sympathetic onlookers are genuine in their concern, and I appreciate their interest in my well-being. Nevertheless, the constant approach and inquiry of strangers can be irritating.

In the past, I would become depressed and withdrawn whenever my odd behavior was questioned. From time to time I would stay at home, feeling too embarrassed to go out in public. A simple task, such as a trip to the grocery store, was a dreaded experience. When the tics were unmanageable, they would draw attention like a magnet.

I have since gotten over some of the fear of ticcing in public, yet continue to be upset at times by the reactions of others. Naturally, I would prefer that my tics not be noticed, and I continue to disguise them whenever possible. Like an "undercover Touretter," an alien among normal citizens, I try not to tic and blow my cover.

There are those less fortunate who are unable to hide their tics at all. They cannot go undercover, and must endure the scorn of others daily. The constant bombardment of disapproving looks, endless questions, and outright harassment eventually becomes unbearable. Sometimes, withdrawal from society seems to be the only viable course of action.

The early years are often the hardest, as Tourettic children sometimes suffer mercilessly at the hands of their peers, who have no understanding of complex neurological disorders. Children simply brand a person who acts differently as an oddball, a good target for teasing.

Numerous horror stories are told of children with tics who are relentlessly tormented by their classmates, making life at school a living hell. For the young, retaliation is only natural. It is not unusual for Tourettic students to end up in trouble for physically attacking their tormentors. This reaction may be extreme, but the anger is understandable.

I often feel the urge to tell judgmental adults to "go to hell." Instead, I usually explain my disorder, giving them an opportunity to learn something about Tourette syndrome. It has been my experience that people who were initially critical may actually appreciate the explanation and grow to accept my tics.

I am fortunate that in my profession, many people seem to accept me the way I am. Being a musician is almost like having a license to act strangely, as artists and musicians have been social misfits throughout history. Wolfgang Amadeus Mozart is believed to have had TS, and Vincent van Gogh was epileptic. Most people seem to embrace such odd behavior as a part of being creative, a characteristic of the quintessential artist.

It is unfortunate that this acceptance does not cross into the business world so easily. Business people frequently have a rigid concept of professional poise, and a person with tics does not fit this image. In the corporate world, being respected is of far greater benefit than being liked.

Due to a fear of losing this essential respect, I avoid business meetings whenever possible, preferring to let someone else handle negotiations. Executives in the recording industry expect an artist to be totally confident and calm, not fidgety and withdrawn. Once a performer becomes famous, the artist's strange behavior is miraculously tolerated, perhaps even viewed as cool or expressive.

These expectations do not exist only in the field of entertainment. Most professions involve some degree of presentation or show, and the performance required by those in other fields is usually more demanding than that of a musician. A corporate executive must appear totally composed at all times in order to avoid suspicions of incompetence. Politicians must seem to have virtually no flaws as humans or leaders.

For those with tics, the inability to exhibit this poise can present a severe handicap, both socially and financially. Although some individuals with TS manage to excel in mainstream professions, most suffer discrimination. Many lose their jobs due to Tourettic behavior. Others are not considered for well-deserved promotions as a result of their humiliating tics.

It is fortunate that many people with TS develop their own effective methods of coping with the disorder. The majority are highly driven individuals, perhaps out of necessity.

Still, a severe case can overpower even the most motivated person, transforming life into a series of miserable, explosive tics. There are many diseases which ravage the body much more severely than Tourette syndrome, but few attack the soul with such vengeance. A patient may be forced to resort to extreme means, such as constant sedation by powerful drugs, or total isolation. In a few cases, distraught TS patients have undergone psychosurgery in a desperate attempt to rid themselves of tics and obsessions. These procedures are controversial, experimental, and at best, extremely risky.

For those with moderate cases, tolerating the disorder is usually less of a problem than dealing with the people who make no attempt to understand it. I am thankful that I have been surrounded by people who do not think negatively of me because of my symptoms. I would much rather have the tics of Tourette syndrome and not be judged for them, than be totally healthy, yet besieged by judgmental people who criticize my every action. Most people would probably feel the same way under similar circumstances.

Imagine attending a quiet lecture while suffering a bad cold, sniffing at least ten times a minute, unable to stop. No medication will help the symptoms, and missing this important event is not an option.

What would bother you the most—the fact that you are sniffing, or the thought that everyone else may be annoyed by your sniffing? I would bet on the latter. Similar uneasiness is experienced by a person with TS every day, every hour, and in every public location.

Relatives, co-workers, and peers sometimes either

lack the intelligence or the humanity to accept tics—many cannot, or will not, understand that inappropriate behavior can be caused by an organic disorder. They assume that if the patient can control tics for short periods of time, he or she should be able to keep them permanently at bay, or at least do so whenever in public. It may appear that the person's tics indicate a lack of self-control and willpower.

It is often forgotten that tics are just as necessary to those with TS as the act of sneezing is to victims of allergy attacks. Most people can hold off a sneeze for a few seconds, maybe longer, but inevitably an uncomfortable sensation will force them to sneeze. The act of giving in to a sneeze does not suggest that the allergy sufferer has no willpower. The same may be said for anyone trying to restrain from vomiting, coughing, or any number of bodily functions. Absolute control is impossible. In the case of tics, the speed and unpredictability with which they occur makes suppression even more difficult.

The Tourettic mind is believed to contain our most primitive animalistic tendencies, emerging in an uninhibited, twisted form. Like a jungle cat quietly waiting to pounce on its prey, the disorder may unexpectedly roar into action at any time, turning a brief moment of tranquility into a nightmare. The psyche of Tourette syndrome possesses at least as much intelligence as its host, and is significantly more cunning. This combination of the primitive and the intelligent causes sudden, explosive, yet complex and sometimes uncouth tics.

Other chemical disturbances, such as intoxication by street drugs or alcohol, can also cause both primitive and uninhibited reactions. The symptoms of TS are different from most of those associated with drunkenness, but the source is nevertheless chemical. The behaviors induced by TS and other disorders, however, do not require the introduction of outside toxins.

The public seems to understand and accept that reprehensible behavior can result from alcohol and drug use, but has difficulty comprehending that it can be caused by built-in imbalances. The self-indulgent drunk is readily forgiven, yet the blameless TS sufferer is shunned.

This lack of understanding applies to many biological conditions. Consider the diabetic who begins to act irrationally during the early stages of diabetic coma. Due to a chemical imbalance, this person temporarily loses control over the mind and body. There are hundreds of documented cases in which people with diabetes were denied medical attention because others assumed that they were drunk from alcohol.

Many of these unfortunate individuals died in hospitals as they awaited emergency treatment.[36]

Just as an imbalance of insulin occurs with diabetes, an imbalance of neurotransmitters causes Tourette syndrome. The two are completely different physical problems, yet both are chemical in origin, and both can produce bizarre symptoms which falsely appear to be either psychologically based or caused by drug abuse. In either case, misinterpretation of outward symptoms can have destructive effects.

Most people with Tourette syndrome do not expect, nor should they, any special treatment. What they should and do expect is to be treated with dignity and equality. Basic human understanding can do wonders to help those with TS, and the lack of it can be devastating, especially to children. Many develop lifelong psychological problems as a result of mistreatment by the people around them.

Perhaps someday the public will learn to accept the tics of Tourette syndrome as easily as they do the sneeze of a common cold. Until then, the old cliché "what you see is what you get" may be the best mode of social interaction for those with TS. With or without tics, a person is either accepted or rejected by others, and must be able to face both possibilities.

Chapter eleven
Final Thoughts on Tourette Syndrome

One afternoon I was having a particularly difficult time with tics while setting up my musical equipment for a performance. A young man approached me with an astonished expression.

"My little cousin does that," he said. "He's been kicked out of school, and his parents have practically disowned him. I'm the only one who will have anything to do with him."

I was struck by feelings of pity for this child, and could not help but feel anger toward his parents and school officials, in spite of their ignorance.

He described his cousin's tics, and I explained that the symptoms sounded like Tourette syndrome. I suggested that he immediately take the boy to see a doctor for a proper diagnosis. I also gave him my phone number, and offered to provide the address of the Tourette Syndrome Association, as well as any other information I could find. I never heard from him again. I hope things worked out well, and this child's disorder is now being properly treated.

While traveling in Italy, I saw a middle-aged man displaying severe motor and vocal tics. He was receiving strange looks from nearby pedestrians as he attempted to gain control and continue moving down the sidewalk. He would take several steps, yelp, and then become frozen in contortions. His arm would flail and his torso would twist. I was upset by this sight and wanted to communicate with him, but I could not speak the language. I also feared that my attempt would cause him additional embarrassment. It was difficult to walk away and do nothing, because I suspected that, like so many others, he may not have had a clue as to the nature of his problem.

Because I am not a doctor or scientist, I feel somewhat powerless to help those who are devastated by this disorder. Perhaps this book will make a small contribution in the battle against TS by waving another distress flag at those who can provide direct assistance.

As TS research continues, scientists will inevitably

create new and better methods for treating the disorder, improving the odds for abatement of symptoms or recovery in even the most severe cases. Although Tourette syndrome's genetic connections to other disorders make it extremely perplexing, these links may eventually prove to be beneficial. Every study of a related condition may provide clues to unravel the TS enigma.

While researchers do biological battle with Tourette syndrome, the average person can help the cause by educating others. One source of the disorder's power is its ability to humiliate and embarrass its victims to the point of ruining their social and professional lives. If the public could become accepting enough to make such humiliation obsolete, a great deal of the disorder's strength would disappear. TS will likely always be a disruptive neurological problem, but it need not be a socioeconomic handicap.

In the real world, people tend to discriminate against any variance from the norm, particularly when they don't understand it or perceive it as threatening. Until this situation improves or a cure is discovered, those with TS must learn to either tolerate or ignore the judgment of others.

The extensive list of symptoms associated with

Tourette syndrome, both direct and peripheral, is continuing to expand, largely because of the growing number of cases studied. Many of these symptoms are variations on similar themes, such as the multitude of obsessive-compulsive behaviors. Others are new and puzzling discoveries. It is easy to become overwhelmed by the number of possible problems which may result from this disorder, yet patients rarely exhibit all of the known symptoms, and many suffer only a few.

Although any disease is an enemy to its victim, Tourette syndrome is rather unique in its ability to whittle away at the sufferer's self image. In contrast to other behavior-altering disorders, TS does not cause a person to lose consciousness or awareness of outside reality. One can never retreat to or become content in a private little world. It is a never-ending struggle to avoid total chaos as the Tourette world clashes with the real one. The battle is exhausting and the casualties are many, including losses in self-esteem, productivity, confidence, and personal relationships.

There is a measure of hope, even for those with the most severe cases. It is estimated that in approximately one-third of all TS patients, the teenage years bring a remission of symptoms. The tics and obsessions may never return. In about half of all other cases, they may not disappear, but significantly decrease by late adolescence.

The remaining patients will probably have symptoms of relatively constant severity throughout life.[37] Even in these cases the disorder is unpredictable and the symptoms may spontaneously improve at any time. TS usually reaches its peak of severity during early adulthood and rarely becomes significantly worse with age. It is far more likely that tics will fade with time.

All of my adult life I have witnessed people who seem to be able to relax and allow their stress to disappear for awhile. They can quietly enjoy a book, drink a cup of coffee with a friend, or watch a movie with no sign of nervous tension. This is just a pleasant part of life that most humans take for granted. Such simple repose is both foreign and truly amazing to me, and I assume it is to others who have TS. As much as we would love to be able to relax, we may never actually realize such an ability.

The only opportunity we have to rest must be purchased in the form of a sedative drug. Without pharmaceuticals we are either focused and working, ticcing, or both. With the help of proper drugs we may reach a state of synthetic relaxation, but only at the price of being dazed from their tranquilizing effects.

To most people, the idea of simple relaxation as a major achievement seems silly. Yet for those of us who live with the onslaught of tics, swimming the English channel is probably a more realistic goal than sitting calmly on a sofa for half an hour.

Even when we are trying to relax, the conflict rages inside the mind, demanding enormous amounts of energy. The rapid-fire of intrusive thoughts, the blitz of urges and obsessions, the tensing of muscles as they launch into frenzies of tics—all of this is exhausting. A person with TS may appear to be sitting calmly, revealing only an occasional twitch or blink; but behind those eyes roars a siege, an electrical storm, a violent confrontation between the understandable and the unthinkable—and so it goes forever.

A person can become so obsessed with Tourette syndrome that it consumes the mind. A developing cycle of obsessions, compulsions, tics, embarrassment, rejection, shame, frustration, and depression can create a whirlpool of despair. Sometimes the only way out of this vortex is simply to ignore the demon whenever possible. To ignore it is to rob it of its power.

I cannot stop the tics and compulsions. They

happen. I perform them—but I try to quickly move on. Goals and dreams come first. I cannot allow the Tourette demon to dominate my thoughts.

Although the disorder causes enormous harm, productive characteristics can result from it. People with TS often excel in creativity, intellect, sports, and musical ability. Although some patients display inferior handwriting skills and other fine motor coordination problems, many exhibit superb reflexes, speed of movement, and agility.

Baseball legend and Tourette patient Jim Eisenreich has become a major spokesperson in the campaign for awareness. His struggle with the disorder and his athletic achievements serve as an inspiration to us all.

Mahmoud Abdul Rauf is an All-American basketball player with TS. Tics did not stop him from setting several NCAA records and becoming a professional ballplayer.

Others throughout history have achieved incredible feats in spite of their obvious tics. Investigators have turned up evidence that Peter the Great and Napoleon Bonaparte, two of history's greatest military leaders, probably suffered from TS. They each rose to power in the days when people with neurological disorders were often locked away or burned at the stake as witches.

Friends and relatives of the great composer Mozart described his eccentric behavior in detail. His actions apparently included a vast array of complex motor and vocal tics, among them, coprographia and coprolalia. He was also well known for his elaborate obsessive-compulsive rituals.

Dr. Samuel Johnson, noted intellect of the 1700's, had a severe case of Tourette syndrome. Johnson is best remembered as a lexicographer and author of *A Dictionary of the English Language*, published in 1755. Several eyewitness accounts recorded by his associates describe the complex details of Dr. Johnson's bizarre ritualistic actions. There was much speculation as to the cause; Tourette syndrome was yet to be identified. In spite of this, Dr. Johnson was greatly admired and became known as "the greatest man of his time."[38]

The same villain which creates internal conflict can provide strength in the external struggle for survival. The world outside may be easier to conquer than the realm of one's own mind.

True inner peace is something people with Tourette syndrome will probably never know. Most of us would give everything we own just to be able to relax, sleep, work, and play without the constant torture of this disorder.

We learn to savor every moment of tranquility life has to offer. During those rare moments, when the demon sleeps, we get a brief, but precious glimpse of serenity.

If you have any questions or comments regarding
the contents of this book, the author and publisher
invite you to send letters and inquiries to:

Silver Run Publications, Inc.
P.O. Box 55
Cashiers, NC 28717-0055

Glossary

This glossary includes several terms which are not found in the text of this book. These additional words, phrases, and expressions have been included because they are relevant to the diagnosis and treatment of Tourette syndrome. For a complete explanation of the following terms, one should consult a physician.

ADD: (see attention deficit disorder)

ADHD: (see attention deficit hyperactivity disorder)

affective disorder: Disorder which affects the mood or

expression of temperament in an individual. Depression is a common affective disorder.

akathisia: Sensation of restlessness; inability to sit still, or feeling that one must constantly move about. This unpleasant sensation often occurs as a side effect of medication.

akinsea: Diminished motor movement or activity. Occurs as a side effect of some medications.

antidepressant: Medication used primarily to control symptoms of depression. Some antidepressants are used to treat other symptoms as well, including those of obsessive-compulsive disorder and Tourette syndrome.

antihypertensive: Drug used primarily to fight high blood pressure (hypertension). Other uses for these drugs have been discovered in recent years. An example is the use of clonidine in the management of Tourette syndrome.

antipsychotics: Group of drugs also known as "neuroleptics," previously called "major tranquilizers." These drugs were developed to treat symptoms of mental illness, but are now used for other purposes as well, including the management of tics.

anxiety: Uncomfortable feelings of uneasiness, apprehension, or fear.

attention deficit disorder (ADD): Disorder characterized by inability to pay attention, tendency to be distracted, and other learning difficulties.

attention deficit hyperactivity disorder (ADHD): Disorder consisting of the learning disabilities of ADD in addition to hyperactivity.

autism: Disorder characterized by extreme withdrawal into one's own world. Symptoms include poor communication abilities, restricted interests, and very poor social interactions.

axon: Fiber of a nerve cell which carries signals to another neuron (nerve cell).

barbiturate: Drug derived from barbituric acid, and used primarily as a sedative or hypnotic. Barbiturates work by depressing the central nervous system.

basal ganglia: Regions of gray matter in the brain which affect both motor function and the transmission of sensory information. These structures are rich in the neurochemical dopamine, and are therefore closely connected to both the occurrence and treatment of disorders such as Tourette syndrome.

biogenic amines: Group of organic chemicals derived from amino acids, which includes the neurotransmitters serotonin, norepinephrine, and dopamine.

bipolar disorder: Current term for manic-depressive disorder.

blood brain barrier: Series of membranes inside the skull which rejects substances in the bloodstream detected to be unsafe to the brain.

central nervous system (CNS): The body's main nervous system comprised of the brain and spinal cord.

chorea: Neurological disorder involving involuntary movements.

clean drugs: Drugs which only affect a specific, targeted system in the body. These drugs produce few side effects, because they do not cause mass changes in brain or body chemistry.

complex tic: Tic which consists of a set or series of movements or vocalizations.

compulsion: Repeated task, behavior, ritual, or act one feels an overwhelming urge to perform. (See obsessive-compulsive disorder.)

coprographia: Involuntary writing of offensive or profane words or statements. A symptom of TS in some sufferers.

coprolalia: Complex vocal tic, occurring in less than a third of all TS patients, in which the sufferer uncontrollably blurts out or shouts offensive or profane words or phrases.

copropraxia: Complex motor tic involving the involuntary making of obscene gestures. Occurs as a symptom of Tourette syndrome in some patients.

dementia: Disturbance of thought processes; loss of intellectual function, orientation, judgment, or memory.

dendrite: Branch of a nerve cell used in the transmission of signals.

depressant: Substance which induces sedation or slows bodily functions.

dopamine: Neurotransmitter involved in movement and other functions. This chemical is closely linked with Tourette syndrome, Parkinson's disease, and other movement disorders.

dysarthria: Difficulty in speech, particularly the articulation of words. May be a side effect of medication, or may result from neurological, psychological, or other physical problems.

dysgraphia: Difficulty with handwriting and associated motor movements. Can occur as a symptom of TS or other neurological disorders.

dyslexia: Reading disorder often characterized by letter or word reversals and spelling errors when writing. May occur as a symptom of TS.

dysphagia: Difficulty in swallowing. Occasional side effect of medication or other medical problems.

dysphoria: Unpleasant state of mood which is often expressed as depression, anxiety, or loss of interest in pleasures.

echolalia: Repetition of the words or sounds of others. A complex vocal tic.

echopraxia: Imitation or repetition of the movements of others. Also called "echokinesis." May occur as a complex motor tic resulting from Tourette syndrome.

EEG: Electroencephalogram. A procedure which measures the electrical activity of the brain.

encopresis: Lack of control of the bowels. Reported as a possible symptom in some cases of TS.

endogenous: Having a biological origin. Tourette syndrome is considered to be an endogenous disorder.

enuresis: Involuntary bed-wetting or lack of bladder control. Unconscious or uncontrolled passage of urine.

enzymes: Substances which bring about chemical reactions.

epilepsy: Disease caused by improper balance of electrical impulses in the brain, often causing convulsive seizures. Although epilepsy is not closely related to Tourette syndrome, the two are sometimes confused.

extrapyramidal effects: Side effects of medication which often involve involuntary movements or motor activities. For example, drugs which effect dopamine levels can cause movements of the mouth and muscle rigidity.

grand mal: Severe seizure accompanied by unconsciousness. A rare, but possible side effect of some medications.

Gts gene: Gilles de la Tourette syndrome gene. The gene (or genes) believed responsible for Tourette syndrome.

half-life: The amount of time it takes for the blood level of a single dose of a drug to fall to half the level of the peak dosage. Useful in determining dosage schedules.

heat intolerance: Excessive discomfort in warm or hot temperatures. Sometimes a symptom of TS.

Huntington's disease (also called "Huntington's Chorea"): Inherited disorder involving involuntary muscle movements, as well as dementia.

hyperactivity (also called "hyperkinesis"): Overactivity. A disorder in which the sufferer cannot sit still and feels the need to be constantly active. Hyperactive children often run and climb excessively.

hypertension: High blood pressure.

hypnotic drugs: Class of drugs used to induce sleep or sedation.

hypotension: Low blood pressure.

kinesthesia: Recognition of movement, weight, strength and position. A disruption of this sense of bodily motion can occur as a side effect of some drugs.

latency period: Period of time before a medication becomes effective.

limbic system: System of structures in the brain which regulates emotions and other thought processes.

lithium carbonate: Drug used to treat many disorders, particularly mania and manic-depressive (bipolar) disorder.

mania: Disorder characterized by high level of excitement.

manic-depression (also called manic-depressive disorder, manic-depressive psychosis or bipolar depression): Disorder characterized by alternate episodes of mania (or excitement, enthusiasm) and depression (or sadness).

mental tic: Tic which involves no vocalization or motor movement. This tic occurs solely in the mind.

monoamine oxidase (MAO) inhibitor: Antidepressant drug which inhibits the action of the enzyme, monoamine oxidase.

mood stabilizing drug: Drug which causes a reduction in mood fluctuation.

motor tic: Involuntary, usually sudden movement of a muscle or group of muscles.

myoclonus: Disorder characterized by spasms or sudden, jerking movements. A twitching or jumping limb is an example of a myoclonic symptom. Myoclonus is an independent disorder, and appears in many people with no other neurological problems. In some cases, myoclonic jerking has been connected to both epilepsy and encephalitis. Some Tourette syndrome patients may exhibit myoclonus, but the two disorders are not considered to be closely related.

neuroleptics: Group of drugs used to treat many disorders, including Tourette syndrome. These drugs are also referred to as "anti-psychotics," or "major tranquilizers."

neuron: Nerve cell.

neurosis: Disorder of the thinking process which does not cause the sufferer to lose significant contact with reality. Examples are anxiety neurosis and hysteria.

neurotransmitter: Chemical which acts as a messenger, carrying signals from one neuron to another.

norepinephrine (also called "noradrenalin"): Neurotransmitter which acts as a modulator of other chemicals in the brain, including dopamine.

nystagmus: Oscillation of the eyeballs. Involuntary, repetitive movement of the eyes. May be a side effect of medication, or may be caused by other medical problems.

obsession: Recurring thought, impulse or mental image. Usually, obsessions are unwanted sensations which repeatedly invade the mind.

obsessive-compulsive disorder (OCD): Disorder characterized by recurring obsessive thoughts and urges (obsessions), and repeated behaviors, performance of tasks, or mental rituals (compulsions). Repeated hand washing is an example of obsessive-compulsive behavior. Often the sufferer will feel an imaginary threat of negative consequences if the ritual is not completed.

oxytocin: Hormone which is involved in contractions during childbirth, and lactation. Also affects grooming and behavior. It is oxytocin's effect on grooming and behavior which heavily connects it to both OCD and Tourette syndrome.

palilalia: The repeating of one's own words. Sometimes a symptom of TS.

panic attacks: Sudden, intense feelings of anxiety which can cause symptoms such as rapid heartbeat and shortness of breath.

Parkinson's disease: Neurological disease which causes a deficiency of dopamine in certain brain cells. Its symptoms include muscle rigidity, tremors, and lack of use of the facial muscles.

PET scan: Positron emission tomography. A medical procedure which constructs a visual image of the brain. This technique is used to study the structure and function of various parts of the brain.

phantom fixation: Mental phenomenon which involves interaction or thought concerning an imaginary (or phantom) object.

phobia: Fear which is experienced in irrational proportions. Common phobias are acrophobia (fear of heights), agoraphobia (fear of open spaces), and arachniphobia (fear of spiders).

phonic tic (also called vocal tic): Involuntary utterance of sounds, words, or phrases.

placebo: Substance which produces no significant effects on the mind or body, often used to create a control group in drug trials.

polydipsia: Excessive drinking of fluids.

psychogenic: Of mental origin. A disorder caused by reaction to traumatic experience is considered to be psychogenic.

psychopathic: Refers to any emotional disorder which results in unusually aggressive or irresponsible behavior. Symptoms may include lack of caring or affection for other people, lack of fear of consequences for criminal acts, or antisocial behavior.

psychopharmacology: The study of medications and their effects on the mind.

psychosis: Mental disorder which includes loss of touch with reality.

psychosomatic symptoms: Symptoms caused by incorrect thinking or emotional disturbance.

psychosurgery: Surgical procedure performed to treat neurological illness with psychiatric symptoms. For example, rare, extreme cases of otherwise untreatable OCD have reportedly been helped by psychosurgery.

psychotic: affected by psychosis.

renal: Refers to the kidneys. Some drugs have side effects which affect the kidneys.

schizophrenia: Illness in which the sufferer exhibits psychotic symptoms, such as hallucinations, delusions, and extremely disorganized thinking.

sedative: Medication which induces calmness or sleep.

serotonin: One of the primary neurotransmitters. Functions of this chemical include the inhibition of inappropriate behavior.

serotonin re-uptake blocker: Antidepressant drug used to treat a number of disorders, including depression and obsessive-compulsive disorder. Also referred to as "serotonin re-uptake inhibitor," and "selective sero-tonin re-uptake inhibitor" (SSRI).

simple tic: tic involving one simple movement or vocal-ization.

synapse: The gap (or junction) between neurons, which neurotransmitters cross in order to carry signals.

syndrome: Group of symptoms which regularly occur together.

Sydenham's chorea: Movement disorder once referred to as "St. Vitus' dance," characterized by uncontrollable muscle movements, and once confused with Tourette syndrome.

tachycardia: Uncommonly rapid heart beat. Approx-imately one hundred beats per minute and over is considered tachycardia. May occur as a side effect of medication, or from other physical problems.

tardive dyskinesia: Literally means "late-occurring difficulty with movement." A symptom which often involves movements of the face (such as chewing movements). Other body parts may be affected as well.

These movements can result from long-term use of some medications.

therapeutic window: The dosage range in which a drug is effective. A larger dosage would result in unacceptable side effects; a smaller dosage would not achieve the desired effect.

tic: Involuntary, sudden, rapid movement, twitch, or vocalization.

tic disorder: Neurological disorder which involves the occurrence of tics. Examples are: transient tic disorder, chronic tic disorder, multiple tic disorder, chronic multiple tic disorder, and Tourette syndrome.

Tourette syndrome (short for Gilles de la Tourette syndrome): Neurological disorder characterized primarily by involuntary movements and vocalizations (motor and vocal tics).

tranquilizers: Group of drugs primarily used to calm or relieve anxiety.

tremor: Involuntary quivering, shaking movement. Tremors may result from a variety of causes, including neurological disorders and the use of certain medications.

tricyclic antidepressants: Group of drugs used to treat depression and other disorders. The term "tricyclic" is derived from the chemical structure of these drugs, which consists of three rings of carbon atoms in each molecule.

tryptophan: Amino acid which is necessary for the manufacture of the neurotransmitter serotonin.

vasopressin (also called antidiuretic hormone): Hormone which performs several functions, including the regulation of urine secretion and blood vessel constriction. Vasopressin is also believed to play a role in grooming and behavior, which links it to both obsessive-compulsive disorder and Tourette syndrome.

vocal tic: Tic involving the vocalization of a word, phrase, or noise. Also called "phonic tic."

APPENDIX A
Pharmaceutical Manufacturers

BRAND NAME ®	MANUFACTURER
Haldol	McNeil.
Luvox	Upjohn
Orap	Gate Pharmaceuticals (US)
	McNeil(Canada)
Ritalin	Ciba
Risperdal	Jannsen
Prolixin	Princeton
Catapres	Boehringer Ingelheim
Luvox	Upjohn
Zoloft	Roerig
Paxil	Smith Kline Beecham
Prozac	Dista
Serzone	Bristol-Myers Squibb
Effexor	Wyeth-Ayerst
Anafranil	Ciba (US)•Geigy (Canada)
Tofranil	Geigy
Norpramin	Merrell Dow
Klonopin	Roche
Valium	Roche
Inderal	Wyeth-Ayerst

NOTE: An excellent discussion of the drugs used to treat TS and related disorders can be found in the book, *A Mind Of Its Own: Tourette Syndrome, A Story And A Guide* (Oxford University Press 1994), by Ruth Bruun, M.D. and Bertel Bruun, M.D.

The Tourette Syndrome Association, Inc. (phone: 718-224-2999) also offers a wealth of information on this subject.

APPENDIX B
Suggested Reading

An Anthropologist On Mars, by Oliver Sacks (Alfred A. Knopf, Inc., New York)

Awakenings, by Oliver Sacks (E.P. Dutton, New York)

The Boy Who Couldn't Stop Washing: The Experience and Treatment of Obsessive-Compulsive Disorder, by Judith L. Rapoport, M.D. (Plume Books, New York)

Children With Tourette Syndrome, A Parent's Guide, edited by Tracy Haerle (Woodbine House, Rockville, MD)

Don't Think About Monkeys - Extraordinary Stories by People with Tourette Syndrome, edited by Adam Ward Seligman and John S. Hilkevich, foreword by Oliver Sacks (Hope Press, Duarte, CA)

Echolalia - An Adult's Story of Tourette Syndrome, by Adam Ward Seligman (Hope Press, Duarte, CA)

Appendix

The Man Who Mistook His Wife For A Hat, by Oliver Sacks (Summit Books, New York)

A Mind Of Its Own: Tourette's Syndrome, A Story and a Guide, by Ruth Dowling Bruun and Bertel Bruun (Oxford University Press, Oxford - New York)

RYAN - A Mother's Story of Her Hyperactive/Tourette Syndrome Child, by Susan Hughes (Hope Press, Duarte, CA)

Tourette Syndrome and Human Behavior, by David E. Comings, M.D. (Hope Press, Duarte, CA)

Teaching The Tiger; A Handbook for Individuals Involved in the Education of Students with Attention Deficit Disorders, Tourette Syndrome or Obsessive-Compulsive Disorder, by Marilyn P. Dornbush, Ph.D. and Sheryl K. Pruitt, M.Ed (Hope Press, Duarte, CA)

Living With Tourette Syndrome, by Elaine Fantle Shimburg (Simon & Shuster, New York)

Children's Books:

Hi, I'm Adam - A Child's Story of Tourette Syndrome, by Adam Buehrens (Hope Press, Duarte, CA)

Adam and the Magic Marble, by Adam and Carol Buehrens (Hope Press, Duarte, CA)

APPENDIX C
For more information

Tourette Syndrome Association, Inc.
42-40 Bell Blvd.
Bayside, NY 11361
(718) 224-2999

CHADD (Children with Attention Deficit Disorders)
499 Northwest 70th Ave., Suite 308
Plantation, FL 33317
(305) 587-3700

Obsessive-Compulsive Information Center
Department of Psychiatry
University of Wisconsin
500 Highland Ave.
Madison, WI 53792
(608) 263-6171

OC (Obsessive-Compulsive) Foundation, Inc.
P.O. Box 9573
New Haven, CT 06535
(203) 878-5669

Appendix

Tourette Syndrome Clinic
City of Hope National Medical Center
1500 E. Duarte Rd.
Duarte, CA 91010
(818) 359-8111

Tourette Syndrome Foundation of Canada
173 Owen Boulevard
Willowdale, Ontario,
Canada M2P 1GA

Manitoba Society for Tourette Syndrome
P.O. Box 25064
1650 Main Street
Winnipeg, Manitoba
Canada R2V 4C7

Tourette Syndrome Association of Australia
Victorian Branch
P.O. Box 86 Bundoora, 3083
Australia
(03) 434-3991 or (03) 459-2748

Norsk Tourette Forening
Christian Melbye
Minkerudasen 33
1165 Oslo 11
Norway
472-285-043

Endnotes

1. Thomas B. Allen, <u>Possessed</u> (New York: Doubleday, 1993) 213.

2. David E. Comings, M.D., <u>Tourette Syndrome And Human Behavior</u> (Duarte, CA : Hope Press, 1990) 685.

3. Ruth Dowling Bruun, M.D. and Bertel Bruun, M.D., <u>A Mind Of Its Own: Tourette's Syndrome, A Story And A Guide</u> (Oxford-New York: Oxford University Press, 1994) 12.

4. Comings, 366.

5. Donald J. Cohen, et al., <u>A Physician's Guide To The Diagnosis and Treatment of Tourette Syndrome</u> (Tourette Syndrome Association, Inc., 1984) 4.

6. Comings, 685-687.

7. Bruce Bower, "Hormone shows link to some obsessions," <u>*Science News*</u>, (29 Oct. 1994): 277.

8. Comings, 685.

9. Teresa G. Allen, BSN, CNP, "Getting Inside: Tourette's Syndrome," <u>*ADVANCE PA*</u> Vol. 2, #10 (Oct. 1994): 11-13.

Endnotes

10. Joseph Bliss, "Sensory Experiences of Gilles de la Tourette Syndrome," Archives of General Psychiatry, vol. 37, (1980): 1343-1347.

11. Cohen, et al., 11, 12.

12. Richard Stickhann, "The Family Tourette," Don't Think About Monkeys, ed. Adam Ward Seligman & John S. Hilkevich, (Duarte, CA: Hope Press, 1992) 102-104.

13. Judith L. Rapoport, M.D., The Boy Who Couldn't Stop Washing (New York: Plume Books, a division of Penguin Books USA Inc.,1990) 118.

14. Allen, 233

15. DSM-IV: Diagnostic and Statistical Manual of Mental Disorders, Fourth Edition. (Washington: American Psychiatric Association,1994) 162.

16. Comings, 115

17. Bliss, 1343-1347.

18. Bruun and Bruun, 68.

19. Comings, 41, 210.

20. Ibid., 314-319, 684.

21. Nancy C. Andreasen, M.D., Ph.D., The Broken Brain (New York: Harper & Row, Publishers, 1984) 132-138.

22. Bower, 277.

23. Rapoport, 219.

Endnotes

24. Physician's Desk Reference (Montvale, NJ: Medical Economics Data Company, 1994) 1357.

25. Allen, 34.

26. Bruun and Bruun, 142-143.

27. Allen, 34.

28. Harold M. Silverman et al., The Pill Book (New York, London: Bantam Books, 1992) 174.

29. Silverman et al., 802.

30. Ibid., 318.

31. Russell A. Barkley, Ph.D., Attention Deficit Hyperactivity Disorder: A Handbook for Diagnosis and Treatment (New York, London: The Guilford Press, 1990) 587-588.

32. Bruun and Bruun, 147.

33. Ruth Bruun, M.D., Commentary on Alternative Therapies for Tourette Syndrome, (Bayside, NY: Tourette Syndrome Association, Inc. Newsletter, Fall-Winter 1983-84)

34. Comings, 250.

35. Ibid., 685.

36. Harvey Grant and Robert Murray, Emergency Care Second Ed. (Bowie, MD: Robert J. Brady Co., a Prentice-Hall Co., 1978) 348.

37. Bruun and Bruun, 45.

38. Ibid., 153-159.

Bibliography

Allen, Teresa G., BSN, CNP. "Getting Inside: Tourette's Syndrome" <u>ADVANCE PA,</u> Oct. 1994: Vol. 2, #10.

Andreasen, Nancy C., M.D., Ph.D. <u>The Broken Brain</u>. New York: Harper & Row, 1984.

Barkley, Russell A., Ph.D. <u>Attention Deficit Hyperactivity Disorder: A Handbook for Diagnosis and Treatment</u>. New York, London: The Guilford Press, 1990.

Bliss, Joseph. " Sensory Experiences of Gilles de la Tourette Syndrome." <u>Archives of General Psychiatry,</u> 1980: 37.

Bower, Bruce. "Hormone shows link to some obsessions." <u>Science News,</u> 29 Oct. 1994

Bruun, Ruth, M.D., "Commentary on Alternative Therapies for Tourette Syndrome." <u>Tourette Syndrome Association, Inc. Newsletter,</u> Fall-Winter 1983-84

Bruun, Ruth Dowling, M.D. and Bertel Bruun, M.D. <u>A Mind Of Its Own: Tourette's Syndrome, A Story And A Guide.</u> London-New York: Oxford University Press, 1994

Cohen, Donald J., et al. <u>A Physician's Guide To The Diagnosis and Treatment of Tourette Syndrome</u>. Bayside, NY: Tourette Syndrome Association, Inc., 1984.

Bibliography

Comings, David E., M.D. <u>Tourette Syndrome And Human Behavior</u>. Duarte, CA: Hope Press, 1990.

<u>DSM-IV: Diagnostic and Statistical Manual of Mental Disorders</u>. 4th ed. Washington: American Psychiatric Association, 1994.

Grant, Harvey and Robert Murray. <u>Emergency Care</u>. 2nd ed. Bowie, MD: Robert J. Brady Co., 1978

<u>Physician's Desk Reference</u>. Montvale, NJ: Medical Economics Data Co., 1994

Rapoport, Judith L., M.D. <u>The Boy Who Couldn't Stop Washing</u>. New York: Plume Books, a division of Penguin Books USA, Inc., 1990

Stickann, Richard. "The Family Tourette." <u>Don't Think About Monkeys</u>. ed. Adam Ward Seligman and John S. Hilkevich. Duarte, CA: Hope Press, 1992

Silverman, Harold M., et al. <u>The Pill Book</u>. New York: Bantam Books, 1992

Index

Index

Index

About the Author

Rick Fowler grew up in the small west Georgia town of Bowdon. He began playing guitar at the age of twelve, and has since performed with several successful bands, touring throughout the United States, Europe, and the Mediterranean.

He was diagnosed with Tourette syndrome at the age of thirty-two. Rick currently resides in Athens, Georgia, where he earns his living as a musician and engineer, both in the studio and on the road.

If you would like additional copies of this book, and are unable to obtain them through your local bookstore, please photocopy and mail in this form.

Silver Run Publications

P.O. Box 6254, Athens, Georgia 30604-6254
Phone : 1-800-563-9193   FAX: (706) 549-7463

Order Form

for

The Unwelcome Companion
An Insider's View of Tourette Syndrome

Price per book: $12.95
PLEASE INCLUDE $2.50 SHIPPING for orders of one book.
Add $1.00 for each additional book.

Number of books ordered: _____($12.95 each)

Shipping: + _____

TOTAL ENCLOSED: $_____

check enclosed ❑   Visa ❑   Mastercard ❑

Card #:_____Exp. date:_____

Signature:_____

SHIP TO: Name and address:

NOTE: For orders in Georgia, please include 5% sales tax

Phone(s): (in case of trouble with delivery):

_____

Customers outside US please send bank check in US dollars, order by credit
card charged in US dollars, or FAX in the order form.